You will be thin and feel great!

Matthew Armstrong

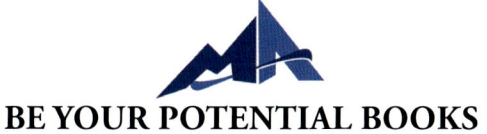

BE YOUR POTENTIAL BOOKS

YOU WILL BE THIN & FEEL GREAT

Published by **Be Your potential**
email: info@beyourpotential.net   Web: http://www.beyourpotential.net To report errors, please send a note to errata@beyourpotential.net

© **Copyright 2008 Matthew Armstrong**

All rights reserved. No part of this work may be reproduced or transmitted in any form by any means, electronic, mechanical, photocopying, recording, or otherwise, without the prior written permission of the publisher. For information on getting permission for reprints and excerpts, contact permissions@beyourpotential.net

The right of Matthew Armstrong to be identified as the author of this work has been asserted by him in accordance with the Copyright, Designs and Patents Act 1988.

British Library Cataloguing in Publication Data
A catalogue record for this book is available from the British Library

ISBN: 978-0-9561713-0-6

Typeset and Graphic Design by Victoria Whitehead
Cover photograph by Yuri Arcurs of Dreamstime.com

Printed and bound in Great Britain

NOTE: The material contained in this book is set out in good faith for general guidance. While every precaution has been taken in the preparation of the book, neither the author nor publisher shall have any liability to any person or entity with respect to any damage or injury caused or alleged to be caused directly or indirectly by the instructions contained in this book.

Contents

Preface — v

Dedication — vii

Acknowledgements — ix

Introduction — xi

Part 1 — The Mind — 15

Part 2 — Nutrition — 67

Part 3 — Exercise — 92

Something fundamental to your success — 122

Transformational Coaching — 125

A final blessing — 126

About the Author — 127

Preface

I would like to share with you my understanding of synchro-destiny. We don't always get what we want, but we do always get what we need. When I sat down to write this book, I was actually going to write a different book, but when I put pen to paper, this is what flowed out. I resisted it, because I had other ideas. After writing about twenty pages and being able to see the whole book clearly in my mind, I said No! closed my writing pad and didn't open it for about a year.

What you resist persists, so finally I couldn't take it any longer and I pulled out my writing pad and gave birth to this book. Through my meditations I was informed that the book that I wanted to write would actually be my third book.

Some people would say that everything is pre-determined in life, and that we are like puppets on a string. Others believe that we have 100% control and that we create our own fate. The understanding I have is that both are working together synchronistically.

To gain a better understanding, let me give you this analogy. When I was learning to drive, I remember that I had control of the car, and I was doing the driving. I was also listening to instructions from the instructor, and as long as I listened and followed what he said, everything went well. One time we were approaching a roundabout, and I made a decision to drive through, even though there were other cars approaching. I ignored my instructors words to stop, as I had already committed myself and thought I was going to make it. He quickly took over and slammed on the brakes, which he had installed in the passenger side for such instances.

In life, this is called divine intervention. We are in control of our lives, and we do have control of our destiny. We also have a guide, that sits with us and walks with us through life. It is up to us to listen and follow their guidance, because they will help us pass the tests. And sometimes they will grab you by the scruff of the neck, sit you down at your desk and then give you some instructions. Do you remember how good it felt when you passed your driving test? It felt good, because it was your hard work that did it, and I will bet that you also thanked your instructor for their expert guidance.

Look at the series of events that guided you to this book, and know that the divine had a part to play in it.

Matthew Armstrong

I dedicate this book to all those who are stepping out from the crowd to bring light to this planet.

Acknowledgements

I was listening to a call-in radio show recently, and the DJ asked the caller if there was anyone he would like to say hello to. The caller said no, because the last time he was on the radio he said hello to a few people and then everybody else he knew hassled him for weeks after because he hadn't mentioned their names.

If I were to thank everyone who helped me arrive at where I am now, with this best-selling book, then it would literally fill another book. If I were just to mention a few people then there would be many who I would miss out.

The truth is, that I thank everyone, even the people who put me down in my life, the people that attacked me, threatened me, abused me, and even the people who tried to kill me, because all of that allowed me the gift of transforming myself and really turning fear into power. It gave me the drive to seek out the master teachers on this planet and learn from them. To take any situation that is now presented to me, give it an empowering meaning, and also be able to say that I have experienced much tougher; even life threatening events, and not just survived, but thrived and was able to grow from them.

So if there's one thing you can take from this book, even before you start reading, it is to be grateful for everyone in your life, past, present and future. Every situation and event, because it is all an opportunity to learn and grow, and all you have to do is ask yourself a simple question; which is "*What can I learn from this and what empowering meaning can I give to this?*" Make this the primary question you ask yourself in challenging times, and it will neutralise all negativity connected to the situation.

When I thank everyone, I also thank you for your curiosity and commitment to living a progressively uplifting life. It is you and all the people you recommended this book to, that is making it into an international best seller, transforming lives worldwide.

With all that said, I would like to thank one more person who has been completely instrumental in taking my scribbled manuscript and presenting it in the form you now have in your hands. She is the love of my life, and is someone who believes in me, even more than I do. Thank you Victoria.

Introduction

Hello and welcome my friend. I would first like to honour and acknowledge you for having the desire and commitment to make massive progress and improvements in your life, and to have the curiosity and openness to attract this book to you and actually read it. You are one of the few who do versus the many who talk, so congratulations.

I wrote this book for you and now I am having a direct conversation with you. You will find that any questions that come to mind as you journey through the pages will be answered later on in the book. There is also a website with video and audio from myself to greatly assist you on your journey all at no extra cost!

I am so very excited for you because this is it! I know that you have had disappointments in the past and each one of those has just brought you closer to the solution that you now hold in your hands. This book is not a tow truck. It is a precise map that when followed correctly will take you to your desired destination, and you still have to do the driving and follow the directions. This is a vitally important distinction.

I am now going to ask you to make four agreements whilst on this journey to ensure your success!

1. Give 100% by being completely honest with yourself.
2. Take notes, highlight, underline and complete exercises.
3. Have fun
4. Share positive learning's with others

If you are not willing to give 100% by being completely honest with yourself, then let me ask you a question! Where else does this show up in your life and what are the consequences for this? Give 100% to this book and it will have a ripple effect into all areas of your life.

When you write things out freehand there is an ingraining of the nervous system, which literally imprints your new empowered choice or belief into your body.

When you have fun and enjoy the journey then there is no resistance and all learning's are received.

When you share your knowledge with others it is very fulfilling and ingrains the learning's even deeper, so you actually embody what you are sharing. Have you ever heard it said, "Teach what you wish to learn"!

If you just read this book passively then you will take in and apply less than 20%. If you read, take notes and complete written exercises then you will take in and apply up to 60%. If you read, take notes, complete written exercises and engage in physiological processes, then you will take in and apply up to 90% of what you could potentially produce in your life from reading this book!

You see this is all about producing results in your life and I would like you to get your moneys worth! Make sense? Great!

Have I got your curiosity yet? Are you excited?
You should be because I guarantee you that this book is like no other you have ever come across. You are about to transform your life! Are you ready?

This is your manual! Write all over it and underline whatever you find most relevant to you. Have your highlighter at the ready for any paragraphs that you resonate with and gives you the greatest distinctions or ah ha moments.

What is very unique to this book and of incredible value, is that you also have an exclusive members website containing audios and videos, which include powerful mind conditioning processes and instructional videos. This is like having me there with you as your personal coach and ensures that you really succeed. It is worth hundreds of times what you paid for this book, and you get it all free, because I want to give you more than you ever expected from me. I also want your results to exceed your wildest dreams. And..they will, when you take advantage of this phenominally powerful resource.

The website is **www.bethinfeelgreat.net** and your password is **believe**.

For you to get the most value out of this I recommend investing one hour a day everyday until you have completed the book including all exercises. Your transformation will take approximately 7 days. Schedule a time everyday when you have no distractions and when you can be by yourself is best. To really own this knowledge to the level where you can teach it, you would spend one hour a day for 21 days, and then there is no going back!

Read and re-read this book. Repetition is so very important. Keep this book with you always and let it be your manual! And your reminder of who you are and how far you have come. Take some before and after pictures of yourself to really make your progress visual! Send them in to me, and if you like I can put them in my next edition!

Now prepare for your transformation! And enjoy the process.

Part 1 – The Mind

"To have willpower is a great start, but to recondition the unconscious mind...then you shall find yourself amongst the stars"
— *Matthew Armstrong*

When you follow all the simple and practical advice that is written in this book, then I have no doubt and I guarantee that you will be thin and look great!

I will make you another guarantee; you will also feel great! And feeling great is what life is all about. And do you know that when you feel great you are unstoppable! You can have, do or be anything or anyone you want, because great feelings attract great things to you. This is the universal law of attraction! Do you get it? Do you want it? How much? Are you willing to open your mind and let go of some disempowering beliefs and install some new powerful beliefs that will change the course of your whole life?

Be willing to open your mind as far as it can go

Are you willing to make some lifestyle improvements? Are you willing to make some new nutritional choices? Are you willing to do new things? Are you willing to make a real commitment to consistent progress in your life?

If your answer to any of these five questions is no, then return this book to me immediately for a full refund, because we would just be wasting each others time otherwise.

You must have spirit and courage for this journey

Still reading? Great! You have spirit and courage and you will need to access your courage more than once throughout this journey that I am now taking you on. I will challenge you on every level. Why? Because it is only through challenge that we evolve, and if you haven't already realised it yet; this book is very special and you have attracted it into your life at this very moment for a very special purpose.

You will be thin, you will look and feel great and a whole lot more...

To state a simple fact. The reason you look the way you look and feel the way you feel is directly related to your daily choices and decisions, which are your habits! You weren't born fat, and it doesn't just run in the family, nor is it in the genes, nor do you have a slow metabolism, or an underactive thyroid. That is all bullshit disempowering beliefs and excuses that will take you no further towards your goals and the results that you want. My outcome is for you to get the result that you are after, and for those results to be lasting. You see I hear those false excuses so often, I thought I would knock them on the head right from the start. You still reading?

Wow... you are tougher than I thought. Like I said. You WILL be thin, and you WILL look and feel great.

You will be thin and you will look and feel great

Many years ago when I ran a gym, I saw a woman totally transform in six months and shed 96 pounds of body fat in that time. The transformation was truly incredible. What I found to be more incredible was that six months after that, she had added another 96 pounds back onto her frame. Back then I really couldn't understand it. It was truly a shame. I completely understood the physical mechanics of how she did it. It was the psychological aspect that mystified me. I am now de-mystified, and so that is what I am sharing with you in this first part. Your mind: how to use it to produce the results in your life that you desire and how fundamentally important this is.

With that said, my first question to you that requires a written answer, is what do you WILL? And before you answer, let me explain to you that your answer needs to be SMART. That is, Stated in the positive, Measurable, Actionable, Realistic and Time driven. I use caution when I say realistic! I mean for you to go beyond what you originally thought possible and for it to be both attainable and sustainable.

If someone else on this planet has done it then it is realistic. Even if no one has, then it can still be realistic.

At the start of 1954 no one had ever run a four minute mile, then Roger Bannister did it. Less than 12 months later, another 7 athletes had run sub four minute miles because they could see that it was realistic. Realistic is in the eye of the beholder. If you believe something is possible with every cell in your body, then it is realistic!

> **If you can dream it, you can do it. Always remember this whole thing was started by a mouse.**
> *– Walt Disney*

Now let me give you an example. "I will weigh one hundred and fifty pounds, I will have twelve percent body fat and I will be able to run six miles without stopping in a time of under one hour. I will have achieved these results within one year."

So this is the one-year outcome, and now lets break that down into three monthly milestones.

THREE-MONTH GOAL
I will shed 15 pounds of body fat and run 2 miles in 20 minutes.

Six-month goal
I will shed another 15 pounds of body fat and run 4 miles in 40 minutes.

Nine-month goal
I will shed another 10 pounds of body fat and increase my distance to five miles in 50 minutes.

Twelve-month goal
I will shed another 10 pounds of body fat, and increase my distance to six miles in sixty minutes.

We have now achieved our outcome!

In the space below, now complete what you WILL, using my example only as a guide, and remember to state everything in the positive!

_____
_____
_____
_____
_____
_____
_____
_____
_____
_____
_____

_____
_____
_____
_____
_____
_____
_____
_____
_____
_____
_____
_____
_____
_____

Now you know what you will, here comes the one that is so very important. Why do you will it? This needs to be extremely compelling; something that creates an emotional charge, and inner drive. Let me give you an example.

"I will achieve these results, because this is who I truly am. My happiness and quality of life will soar. I will be able to walk along the beach in a swimsuit or shorts and feel confident. My new self will positively affect all those that I come into contact with".

Your new self will positively affect all those you come into contact with

Write as much as possible because the bigger your WHY is, the more drive you will have to complete your goals and blast through any obstacles!

In the space provided below, now complete your WHY.

_____
_____
_____
_____
_____
_____
_____
_____
_____
_____
_____
_____
_____

If your compelling WHY is to impress a guy or girl you like, or to please your friends, go back and do it again, because such reasons are very often short lived, and it puts you at the effect rather than at cause. Which means, if you fall out with the guy, or your friends then it will give you an excuse to quit. We shall talk more about being at cause shortly.

What must happen now before you turn the page, is that you need to take an action towards the attainment of your goal. Remember you are at cause, so I am not going to tell you what to do, because then you would be at the affect of me, and I want you to use and further develop your decision making muscles and your creativity.

I shall give you a few examples of what immediate action you could take.

1. Activate your free membership at www.bethinfeelgreat.net (Remember, your password is "Believe").
2. Make yourself a large plate of salad and raw vegetables and eat the lot.
3. Write your shopping list and make 50% of it vegetables.
4. Go onto www.bethinfeelgreat.net and order your discounted high quality juicer.

I recommend doing all these things. Right now, just do something, get the ball rolling, because once it does, you won't want to stop. You can do whatever you will, just do something. Now seriously take action right now before you turn the page, because if you don't, then you won't do anything; I mean it, stand up right now, take a deep breath in and shout Yes, whilst punching your fist in the air, and take action NOW. I believe in you.

See you when you get back.

If for some excuse (*because there are no reasons just excuses!*) you didn't take action then please read no further, because this book and course really isn't for you. Give it to someone who is going to get value from it, because you have just wasted your time and money. Do it now!

You are still reading, so well done. How does it feel? Easy wasn't it, once you made that decision. This is what it feels like to be empowered and in control of your life. Our decisions shape our lives.

Our decisions shape our lives

Indecision is a decision. This is really the power that you have. I am sure you know all this already, and quite often we know what to do and don't do what we know. It is the awareness that you are in control, that you are at cause, and you can shape your body, your mind, and your life in any way you wish. As the genie says "your wish is my command" and the genie is in each and every one of us. Become aware of this and use it. This is power my friend.

Now when we get right down to it, right down to why in the past you haven't been totally happy with your appearance. It's because of your thoughts. Your thoughts are the root cause of where you are right now in your life. Change your thoughts and everything will change. The sequence goes as follows.

THOUGHTS lead to FEELINGS, which lead to ACTION or INACTION, which produce your results.

This is why the first section of this book is dedicated to the internal game. Because when the mental, emotional and spiritual aspects get handled, then the physical part is easy and effortless. In fact the physical is actually a manifestation of the mental, emotional and spiritual, so put the effort in now!

Do the mind conditioning exercises, and read and re-read until you take all this information in beyond intellectually, and internalise it so every cell of your body understands and is in agreement.

When we put our attention on something, we get more of it. Even when I say *"I wish I wasn't so out of shape"* By thinking about that, I will become more out of shape, because the unconscious mind cannot process negatives. What it hears is *"I wish I was so out of shape"* Try this one instead *"I wish to be in phenomenal shape"* Say this continuously and feel how it resonates in you. Now realise this; where attention goes, energy flows. Understand!

The unconscious mind can't process negatives

An exercise that we are now going to do is to put our attention on all that we are and all that we have, basically everything in our life that we are grateful for. So to start with right down 25 things, that you are grateful for, and it will be easy to skip right past this and say I will just read it first and then go back and do the exercises. Procrastination is the silent assassin, and you must be prepared to change that right now. Start living in the moment, because this is your life!

Gratitude is your catalyst to happiness

You are exchanging time, which is the most precious resource you have, to read this book. There is a reason I say to do things a certain way, and it is so you can produce results and make consistent progress in realising your dreams, that will alter your whole existence for the better, and that is to have the body that you will and deserve. Remember, that is just the physical reward. The invisible rewards are immeasurable. The universe rewards those who feel grateful.

The Universe rewards those who feel grateful

Make that list now!

25 THINGS I AM GRATEFUL FOR RIGHT NOW:

_____
_____
_____
_____
_____
_____
_____
_____
_____
_____
_____
_____
_____
_____
_____
_____
_____

_____

_____

_____

_____

_____

_____

You did it, great! How was it? A question I have, is was it an intellectual process, or did you really feel gratitude when you wrote each one down. The important thing is that you did it. And the more you do it, the more you will feel it. And as I have said, what you put your attention on, you get more of. So doing this process often, like every day means that more and more things that you could be grateful for will flood into your life. You don't have to take my word for this stuff, its the law. Not a law that is created by the government and enforced by the police, because if it was, then maybe we would have world peace. This is the universal law of attraction. What we focus on with emotional intensity, we bring into our lives. What we think, what we say and what we do, in other words, thought, word and deed. This is reality.

With this understanding, you can shape your body to how you will it. You can even shape your facial features. And even bigger than that, you can shape your destiny, and existence on our planet as we know it. You see I want to tell you, that you are a wonderful powerful being, a human being, which is the most powerful of all the beings on planet earth, and that we know of in existence. Your potential is so vast and huge, and all the other big words a person can think of, that to comprehend we would have to understand where infinity finally ends.

Energy and persistence conquers all things
– Benjamin Franklin

All we must understand is that there is no limit to it. You WILL be thin, and you WILL feel great. Believe that right now and the rest will take care of itself. You must be willing to do whatever it takes.

Put your hand on your heart right now and say three times... *"I will do whatever it takes to get myself in phenomenal shape"* What is phenomenal shape? People's ideas of this differ greatly. So this brings us onto visualisation. You must have a picture in your head of exactly how you desire to be and look. It needs to be a detailed image of exactly how you look, what clothes are you wearing because of your new look, and all the confidence that goes along with it. How do you stand? What is your posture like? How do you gesture? When you speak, how does it sound? Is your voice more resonant? What sort of expression is on your face? Are you smiling? Is there a new determination in your eyes? How do you feel? Is there a new found sense of accomplishment within you?

You may feel a great deal more secure and confident within yourself. How does everyone else around you respond to you? Possibly you are receiving more respect and admiration? How is the opposite sex now attracted to you? How has your life changed and progressed?

These are all things to take into consideration when visualising the new you.

I hear and I forget, I see and I remember, I do and I understand
— *Confucius*

Now stand up! Yes right now... Stand up! If for some reason you can't, like you are on public transport, then save this process until you get home. Just make sure that you do it.

Go to **www.bethinfeelgreat.net** and play Audio 1.

So you are now stood up, right? Make sure that there is a space of at least two foot in front of you. Do this first with your eyes open so that you can read it, then do it again afterwards with your eyes closed, and it will be even more powerful. Bring up the image of the desired new you now. Maybe it is six months from now, or a year. See yourself vibrant, healthy, happy, and every little detail that you can picture. As you think of more things. The picture becomes brighter and brighter and more and more intense. And now the new you is standing directly in front of you with their back to you. And now you step right into the new you, and actually step forward into your new body.

You are now in the picture, you are there, you have done it. Because when you go there in the mind, you will go there in the body. Congratulations.

The power of visualisation should never be underestimated. All great people in history understood this and used it. When Andre Agassi was once asked how he won Wimbledon, (*the most prestigious tennis event in the world*), he simply said, "*It was easy, I had already won it thousands of times in my head"*.

Always start with the end in mind. Every invention, building, film and book that ever existed, was first a vision inside someone's head, which they believed in and consistently focused on until it became manifest. Your body is no different.

There are two things that stop people from getting what they really want. Before I state them, I will let you know that these things don't apply to you, because you are a warrior.

The two things that stop *other people* from getting what they want are:

Firstly, Excuses – Tell me what excuses did you used to use that prevented you from getting what you want. A common one is, "*I've tried everything and I just can't lose weight.*" My question would then be… "*Everything?*"

And the answer to that is of course No, because there is always something that will work if you keep on keeping on.

If we all did the things we are capable of, we would literally astound ourselves.
– *Thomas Edison*

After 9000 experiments and attempts to create the electric light bulb, Thomas Edison, didn't say, "I've tried everything, and it's just not working" Although he had a right to. It was his amazing psychology that propelled him forward to finally crack the code after over ten thousand attempts. And that is the single most important thing you must develop, for you to get to where you are now heading. "*What's that?*" You ask. "*An amazing psychology of course.*" That is to have total unwavering belief in yourself. You are now starting to realise, that there really are no excuses. What a person is really saying when they make an excuse of why they aren't achieving their desired goal or intention, is that they just aren't willing to do whatever it takes. Decide that you are willing to do whatever it takes! Let go of those old stories now, and feel yourself being magnetically pulled, progressively towards the new you.

Decide that you are willing to do whatever it takes

The second thing that stops people from getting what they want is Self-Sabotage. "What's that?" again you ask... Well Self- Sabotage is rife in nearly every human being alive. It is unconscious and can be a tricky one, because it hides in the shadows of your unconscious mind. Self-sabotage is actually a protection mechanism installed in the unconscious mind usually as a child to protect you from harm. The only thing is, now it no longer serves you in a positive way.

Self-sabotage usually shows up as disempowering beliefs and also beliefs that conflict with that of the conscious mind, thus creating resistance. For example, if a person runs a business and is seemingly doing their best to make that business a success by bringing in lots of money. But as a child they had a strong religious upbringing and regularly heard statements such as "money is the root of all evil", or "a rich man can no more get into heaven than a camel pass through the eye of a needle". These will be implanted in their unconscious mind and no matter how hard they try to build their business, it won't work out because they will be unconsciously sabotaging themselves on their way and won't consciously understand why.

And you know what! Nothing has any meaning except the meaning we give it! So when an obviously broke person says to me that rich man, camel, needle, heaven thing, I explain that the meaning is that you should use your money for good while you are here because you can't take any material wealth with you. Simple!

"No one was ever thin in our family, being big is in the genes and it just can't be helped"

If a person heard a family member say this repeatedly when they were a child then it would stick in the unconscious mind and would become part of their identity. Even if consciously they felt uncomfortable about being overweight, the unconscious mind would say *"it's OK, it's just who you are, and you can't do anything about it."* That is what is called a disempowering belief, because it strips the person of any power to do anything about it.

The truth is, that we are the most powerful beings in this universe that we are aware of. Out of the billions of living species, none even come close to how powerful we human beings are. And at the moment, most people are only using a minute amount of that power. Really only because

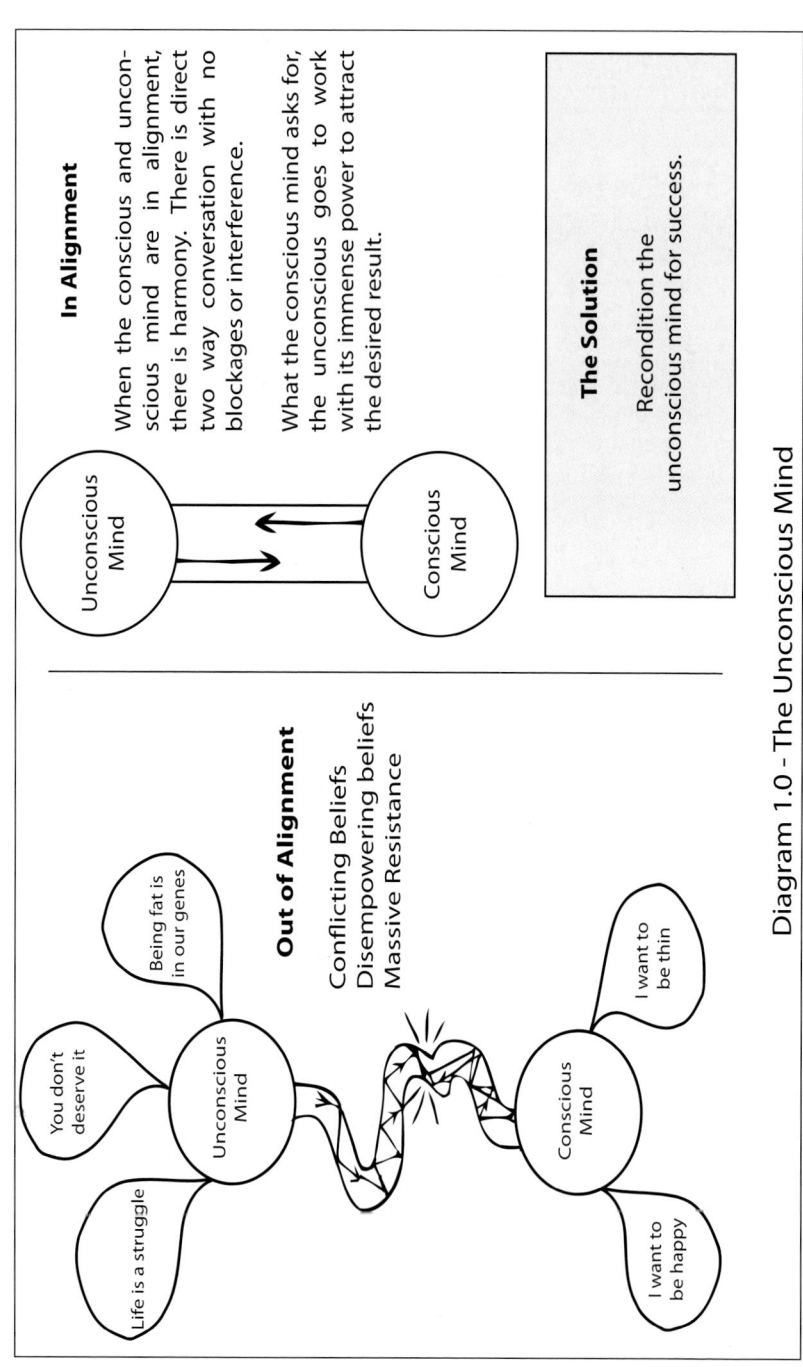

Diagram 1.0 - The Unconscious Mind

they haven't realised the other 99.?% is there. It's always been there.

When a belief in the conscious mind becomes so certain, it starts to dissolve the disempowering ones in the unconscious. One way to do this is through saying a mantra over and over again. There is one that I will give you here, which is in strict accordance with the truth. *"I am whole, perfect, strong, powerful, loving, harmonious and happy."*

Stand up right now, and start to chant this mantra over and over for two minutes. If you are in a public place people might get freaked out, so use discretion. Make sure it's a strong resonant voice, and that you really feel it and mean it. This is the path of self-love. This is the only path. When you can put your hand on your heart, which is right now and say, I truly love myself, go ahead do it. Then my friend, you have nothing to be concerned about. If you just had trouble doing that or didn't even entertain the idea, then you know that you really need to start, seriously. If you found yourself nodding your head back and forth when you did that, then you can be sure that your unconscious mind is in agreement.

Feeling good is the internal key to attracting into your life that, who you truly are, and the environment, which supports that

There are three things that dictate whether we feel good at any particular time. And guess what...You are in control of these three things.

The first is our physiology, and that is anything we do with our body including breathing, gestures etc.

If I wanted to feel depressed, that would be easy. All I would have to do is slump my shoulders forward, drop my head, and shallow breathe into the top of my chest while frowning!

If I wanted to feel relaxed and peaceful, I could lie flat on my back, and relax all my muscles and do some deep diaphragmic breathing with a gentle smile on my face.

To give you an example of just how powerful a shift in physiology can be to change how you feel in an instant, a friend of mine came to me who was experiencing some major life challenges (*from his perspective*). He told me that he was seriously contemplating suicide. At that point I said "*no problem let me straighten you out, turn around*" and I gave him a chiropractic adjustment aligning his spine and pulling back his shoulders. Crack, crack, crack, crack. "*Wow, what was I talking about there, forget I said anything. Let's go and get some lunch*" Were the next words to come out of his mouth. He never brought up the subject again. A slight shift in physiology can totally shift the way you feel, and you can see how the change in physiology then had a knock-on effect with his focus and the language he was using.

This now brings us to the second thing that determines how we feel at any time, which is our focus. Anything we put our attention on affects how we feel. Switch on the news, and you will be bombarded with all the terrible things that are happening in the world. Now flick it over to the comedy channel and watch your mood change. Focus on everything that you are grateful for and by the universal law of attraction, more things to be grateful for will start appearing in your life. This is how powerful your focus is. What you focus on expands.

The third is language. This is what we say outwardly and also the internal self talk.   If you are constantly saying, "*I can't lose weight, I can't lose weight*" The universe will give you just that, which is not losing weight.

If you say "*I am a fat person*" That will have a totally different affect on your mind and body than if you were to say, "*I am in the process of releasing some weight*" This is because saying "*I am a fat person*" makes being fat, a part of your identity.

And here's one of the great secrets of life:

The single biggest motivator in the human psyche is for one to stay congruent with one's own identity

Meaning, if you see yourself as a fat person, as opposed to someone with a little bit of extra weight on, then you will do anything to stay a fat person. Because it is who you believe you are. So this is how important it is to be mindful of our language, what we say out loud, and also the little stories that go on inside the head.
One day, there was a little frog, sitting on the riverbank minding his own business when he was approached by a

scorpion. The scorpion asked the frog to carry him on his back across the river. The frog said *"But you are a scorpion and scorpions sting frogs. If I were to let you on my back and bring you across the river then you would surely sting me."* The scorpion laughed and said *"Don't be silly little frog, if I were to sting you then you would die and I would drown too."* The frog seeing the logic in what the scorpion had said agreed to carry the scorpion across the river. The scorpion crawls onto the frogs back and the frog starts swimming across the river. Sure enough about mid-stream the scorpion, unable to resist any longer, stings the frog. The frog in amazement says *"Why did you do it Mr Scorpion, I will die, and you shall drown too."* *"Well little frog"* replied the scorpion *"That is true, but I am a scorpion, and that's what scorpions do! They sting little frogs."*

We are not scorpions, we are humans, and can change our identity at will. This is the freedom we have. So let's stick with language for now, and the power that our words have. The sentence "I am fat" is more powerful than the sentence "I will be thin". Grouped together, the two words "I am" are the most powerful and influential words we as humans have. So if you've been saying to yourself, in your head or out loud. "I am fat" over and over again, for many years. Then replacing them with the words " I will be thin" Sounds very positive, but just isn't going to cut it!.

You must BE that which you wish to be

There is no someday, there is only now. Be it in your mind, and your body and all around you will follow.

I AM THIN AND I DO FEEL GREAT!

Gandhi understood this great truth when he said *"Be the change you wish to see in the world"*

Be the change you wish to see in yourself

I say "Be the change, you wish to see in yourself".

You must shift your consciousness now to deciding and then realising that you already are, who and what you wish to be.

If you saw this book with this title you more than likely wouldn't buy it. Because you would have thought that it does not apply to you. Well, as you now transform so does the title of your book! This is fun and exciting and you must do it.

Now colour in the text on page 37, cut it out, and use some Pritt Stick to glue it onto the front cover. As you do this, become really excited, remember back to when you were very young at school and you would cut things out and stick them onto something you were creating. **THIS IS IDENTITY CREATION.** The physical action of doing this will create a shift in your unconscious mind, transforming your identity. Remember, thought word and deed. You think it, you say it and you do it. This is true power. Make sure you do this now to complete the circuit. Your new mantra is. *"I am thin and I do feel great"*.

Say it over and over with a big smile on your face, and keep saying it, until you really feel it and every cell in your body is in agreement. This is a powerful manifestation process.

Seeing is not believing; believing is seeing.

Become a leader right now! A leader of your thoughts, a leader of your emotions, a leader of your physical actions. True leaders lead themselves first. They take charge of their thoughts, their emotions, their actions and hold no-one else responsible but themselves. Choose to lead your life this very second and everything will change. If you haven't already worked out what this book is about, then it is about transforming your identity from who you thought you were, to who you are at your core and in your heart.

When I was eleven years of age, I wasn't really aware of how skinny I was. There was a photograph taken of me at a water park and I was shocked to be able to see each individual rib protruding up to my collar bone. That weekend I went shopping with my mother and came back with a large poster of Arnold Schwarzenegger (from the film Commando), and two dumbbells. I pumped those dumbbells everyday while looking at the poster. Then in my mid-teens I realised that I didn't have the bone structure or genetics to sculpt my body into that shape and I didn't really want to either, as I was a martial artist and not a body builder. So the new image I put up on my wall was Jean-Claude Van Damme. We were very similar height, bone structure and were both martial artists. Interestingly enough, I developed a physique similar to Van Damme's and became a Commando in the Royal Marines. Never underestimate the power of continued focus and visualisation.

Dig out the most unflattering photo of yourself and let it be the kick up the backside you need to spur you into action.

Grab some magazines and cut out someone with the body that you desire, or go out or on-line and purchase a poster of someone with the body that you wish to have. Like I was, be somewhat realistic so if you do have a big bone structure, then choose someone who has a big bone structure and is in great shape. Also be careful what is written on the poster, because that could come true as well! Put it somewhere you will see everyday and focus on it with positive intention.

We are now going to do some weeding, of the mind that is. Think of your mind as a garden. Some people work on their garden every day. They might also invest a great deal of money in their garden. Creating water features, bridges, stonework, beautiful flowers and shrubs. They cut the grass and weed it regularly. While others take no care of their garden at all. It becomes overgrown, more and more weeds grow with deeper and deeper roots. Other people around that person can see that they don't respect their garden, so in turn they don't either. They dump their rubbish in it, and persuade their dog to crap in it, so they don't have to clean it up. It is not a pleasant place to be, and the owner of the garden doesn't like to spend much time there. They distract themselves with other activities so they don't have to focus on their mind... I mean their garden. The people with the beautiful Zen minds...or gardens love to spend time there, as it is a very pleasant place to be.

Your garden is your mind, and your mind is your garden. What you do or do not do with it is your choice. If you have never worked on your mind in such a way then be ready for an adventure, because this process is fun and more satisfying long term than anything.

There are three weeds in our garden, which we must take firmly by the roots and toss them out of our mind. Clearing these weeds will give us back control of our minds and our lives.

The first is blaming. By blaming we are not taking responsibility for ourselves, our actions or anything that happens to us. *"It's not my fault I'm fat, it runs in my family"*, or *"my mum fed me too much when I was a child and now I'm just stuck that way"*, or *"my partner put too much pressure on me to lose weight and that just makes me want to eat more"*. These are all ways to blame something or someone else outside of the self to take the pressure off yourself, so that it is not your responsibility. I say take total responsibility now. Even if you don't feel responsible. Take responsibility as it will serve you, and not taking responsibility will not. I often say to my clients who refuse to take any responsibility for their actions, *"Who is in control, if not you? Who is making you eat that doughnut or extra portion, or who is stopping you from going for a run?"*

"Does that person have a control pad and just press buttons when they want you to do or not do something? Explain to me exactly how it works. So if I wanted someone to make me overeat, how would I do that?"

I actually make it sound so silly and irrational, (because it is) that the client makes a shift and moves from a place called

being at the effect of other people, events, situations and experiences, to **being at cause.** Where they realise that no-one is in control but them, and they can choose their life having the greatest freedom of being able to choose their attitude in any given situation. This is really juicy stuff, so I recommend reading it a few times, highlighting your distinctions.

I now invite you to close your eyes. Not yet! And see that blaming weed, protruding out of your head. You may only have a small weed, whilst others will have larger ones.
Grab that weed at it's base, uproot it, and toss it away. Close your eyes and do it now. Easy huh. Well it is something that you must be constantly aware of so that it never returns.

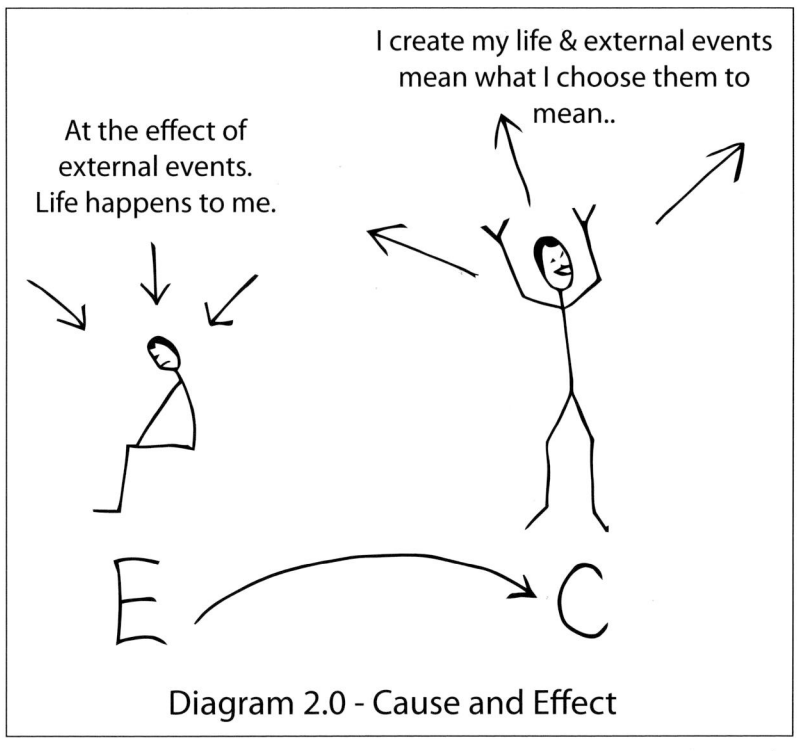

Diagram 2.0 - Cause and Effect

The second weed is complaining. You cannot complain and be grateful at the same time. Complaining has a negative and a debilitating effect on us and some people are experts at it, because it is what they focus on. They always get more things to complain about, and what they focus on expands and is attracted into their life. And while they attract things to complain about, then there is no room for the good stuff. Complaining is also highly infectious like an airborne disease, so I recommend staying clear of complainers.

This is what a complainer will say who "wants" to get in shape. "*No diet I try works. I am so fat and I can't find any clothes that will fit me, and I will never find my soul mate.*" This is the place of the victim, and this attitude and frame of mind is far uglier, than they could ever possibly imagine themselves physically.

There are no ugly people, only ugly attitudes

An attitude can be changed in a heartbeat, or at the speed of thought. Now close your eyes, reach up and take that complaining weed firmly at its base and pull it out watching all the roots come out with it, and now toss it away.

The third weed is rationalising, and this is the smartest of the three because it will rationalise how you are not blaming, complaining or even rationalising. Or if it can't do that, it will rationalise how it is OK to rationalise, blame or complain in certain situations. Do not be fooled by it. It will lower your standards and your potential to achieve your hearts desires will lie dormant.

This weed will come up with all the reasons, (*another name for excuses*) why you can't take action or follow through. Why you have to stay in the job that is not in alignment with your true self. The clues are often in the language. If a client says to me "*Well I just couldn't stick to my nutritional plan last week, because we had relatives staying, and I had to eat what they were eating and they liked to stay up late and I had to get my eight hours sleep so I couldn't get up early to exercise.*" The words *Had, have* and *couldn't*" are clues.

Get on purpose. Get in flow, and then there is nothing you have to do. You GET to do a great many things. Have-to is an illusion. There is nothing you have to do.

The rationalising weed generally butts in about now and says "But I have to pay my bills, if I don't then I'm out on the street". You don't have to. You GET to. Paying bills is a great opportunity to give back for what you have received. This is a co-operative flow of energy in accordance with nature's laws. If I hold onto what I receive and don't give back, or give back begrudgingly, then I am still holding on and the energy is blocked, becomes stagnant and I get fat. This slight shift in focus and in attitude changes everything. Is this making sense? I trust that it is, because it is vitally important that you understand this. It will change everything. The understanding of this and the application of it will change your life.
Being totally honest with yourself, cutting out the BS, will free you of the rationalisation weed. Now close your eyes,

reach up and grab that rationalising weed. Don't rationalise yourself out of doing it by saying I will do it later, or I don't need to take the physical action. Just do it now. Grab it tightly and pull it right out of your head. You will see the very last root come out, and now toss it away.

Go to **www.bethinfeelgreat.net** and play audio 2

Congratulations, and well done. You can celebrate by putting on some lively music and dancing around your house. Seriously lively music and dance!

Feeling good now? Great!

By removing those three weeds from your mind and committing to keeping them out puts you in the top one percent of the worlds population as regards to having an amazing attitude. Your standards are now higher than probably anyone you know. To stop those weeds from creeping back in, you must be vigilant, guard your mind and if one pops up from time to time, don't beat yourself up over it. Instead like the master tending his Zen-Garden say "*Oh, a weed, I must pull that out*". You see it's all about creating habits. Freeing ourselves from habits that do not serve or support us, and replacing them with habits that do. The habits of the mind manifest in the body and in our actions and inactions. And that is why we must tend to our mind first, and the rest will take care of itself.

What we are really doing here is getting rid of all possible excuses, effectively letting go of our story. Our story of why we can't be thin, why we can't be happy and why we can't live the life of our dreams. These are all stories that we tell ourselves. Now release any stories that may be holding you back. Release them right now, and breathe in the freedom that it brings knowing that nothing can stop you! You are on purpose, and you are thin, toned and you do look and feel great.

Let this now be your new mantra. "I am thin, and I look and feel great." Say this often, say it emphatically, and say it like you mean it. Let it be your truth that vibrates from the core of your being, from the depths of your heart and soul and let it manifest into your physical reality. Be aware that you need not make anything happen. When you align with your true self, this is called allowing. Everything you could possibly ever dream of wanting in your entire life, is already there waiting for you to allow it to come into this dimension.

Quite often when a person tries to make something happen in their life, they actually push it away. It is like the little boy who wants to pick up the ball, but every time he runs up to it, just before he can reach it, his foot accidentally kicks it away, and he keeps trying to make it happen, and in his haste, keeps kicking it away. The life of your dreams is already here right in front of you. All you have to do is start to vibrate at the same frequency as what it is you want and it will appear before your eyes, and all around you, and you will hear, see feel and know that your destiny is to BE YOU. Be thyself and know thyself.

Be thyself and know thyself

This is your destiny and this is why you are here. I don't know exactly who you are and exactly what you want. What I do know is that your true self is a fit, healthy, vital and energetic person. And anyone who says that is not what they truly want is deluding themselves. I am glad this is not you. Take hold and open up to your destiny. Let it into your life. The rewards are infinite and the consequences for not doing so are not worth focusing on...or are they?

Go to **www.bethinfeelgreat.net** and play Audio 3
(*To really achieve full value from this next process, you must visit the web site and listen to audio 3.*)

We are now going to go through a little process using the universal law of Polarity, which will be somewhat painful for a few minutes, and I challenge you to stick with it, because it will create a powerful energetic shift within you, catapulting you forward to produce profound results in your life.

I want you to imagine, that you decided that I was full of it, and you weren't going to read another page. In fact, you are going to throw this book in the bin and decide that it all seems like too much hard work and you want the easy life... so you don't change. You just keep going in the direction you were going before you picked up this book, and imagine yourself six months from now. How is your life? How are your relationships? What is your body like? What is your health like and how are your emotions and self esteem because of it.?
Close your eyes for 30 seconds and imagine your life and its downward spiral as you become more unhealthy, fat and out

of shape, Mentally, emotionally and physically.

Now go five years in the future and see how you have deteriorated in all areas of your life. Because how you look and feel affects everything. After five years, how fat have you become? What do you look like? How much pain are you in physically, mentally and emotionally? What are your relationships like, and who has suffered because of you?

What about your career, how has that suffered, because you weren't willing to step up and make a shift in your life. But even after seeing all this you still don't change!

Now close you eyes for another 30 seconds and really visualise this happening. See it, hear it, smell the stench of it and feel the heavy fearful feelings surrounding it. Do it now!

Not finished yet...

Now go 10 years into the future. Where your life has deteriorated so badly it is just disgusting. How grotesque have you become? What is your emotional state like? How much has your self-esteem plummeted? How has your life fallen down around you? Where have your relationships gone? What has happened to your health? How much pain are you in? How much do you regret throwing that book in the bin!

But you can't change, because now you go to an unspecified time in the future and as you look around you realise that you are at a funeral and you are in line to walk past the open coffin, and as you walk past you look down inside and it is you. Lying dead in the coffin, and it is your funeral. And as you walk around, you see a few friends and family and they are saying: If only you had taken care of yourself a little better, you wouldn't have died in such pain and agony. Because your health issues mounted up over the years, you became more obese and dis-ease proliferated throughout your mind and body.

Are you now ready to change, because this is your life? One chance, one opportunity to change it all. To take total control over your future and ultimately your destiny. Come right back to now and realise that now is the time. There is no other time only now, and you are the one who decides what happens and what direction your life takes. So now stand up and take a deep breath shout out the first thing that comes to mind. Punch your fist in the air, clap your hands as you now take charge of your destiny.

This next part can be done standing. Now go one year into the future. Where you have made the changes, you have taken the actions and see yourself, the new you...How do you feel? What is your energy like? How do you look? How have you changed physically? Who do you love? Who loves you? What great things are people saying to you about the new you? What beautiful scents can you smell in the air? How much admiration do you now have for yourself? And see how other people now look at you and the respect and admiration they now have for you. What expression do you have on your face? How happy are you? How full of joy, and how peaceful do you feel?

Step into the new you now, and become that person. BE who you truly are. You are now going to flood your whole body with these positive emotions and experiences. As you stand there glowing with energy, you now reach out your arms in front of you and start to pull in every great experience achievement, and moment in your life from the past, present and future moments. Pulling them into your heart. Pull your hands in and then reach out again and pull another one in, and another, and another. And keep going getting faster and faster flooding your body with positive emotion, all the joy, all the fun all the laughter, all the love. And move right through the present, into the future and all your goals, all your hearts desires, you have achieved them, and as you do this chant "Yes, Yes, Yes" over and over as your body fills with Joy, Happiness, Excitement, Fun, Laughter and finally stand there still and breathe in the peace and feel it all around you. Feel the stillness, experience total peace inside and outside of you, and now the inside and outside blending into one.

This is who you really and truly are. When you come to this space. This is your true authentic identity.

Congratulations my friend, you have just transformed yourself at the cellular level and you are now basking in a sea of potential.

In this great state and feeling all these great feelings, take five minutes to write down your new identity, which you will live by from this day forward. Use the whole page if you can.

Remember what I shared with you earlier, that the biggest motivator in human behaviour is to be congruent with ones own identity. That is, your daily actions will support and be in alignment with your identity. The reason that it is the biggest motivator is because it actually takes no motivation at all. It is just who you are. A smoker doesn't have to pump himself up and push himself to have a cigarette. He is actually on autopilot when he does. And when he doesn't get to have a cigarette for whatever reason, he becomes uncomfortable, because his identity is that of a smoker.

One of my martial arts students, who had been training with me for over 6 months, wasn't able to train with me for a week due to other commitments. He became very uncomfortable and slightly anxious that week. He told me this and I explained to him that it was a great thing, because now he saw his identity as being a martial artist and now he needs more motivation not to train than to train.

So you see, it not about motivation, its about creating an Identity for yourself that serves you at your highest level. Again, if you saw yourself in the past as a fat person, then you would have done anything to stay congruent with that identity at an unconscious level. Even though consciously it was causing you a lot of pain.

Now, you must create habits that are congruent with your new identity. Have another look now at the identity, which you have just created for yourself and if there is anything else that you want to add, then do so. And anything that you want to take out, then do that.
Your daily actions from now on, will start to condition this new identity in, I am not saying that it will be a walk in

the park. You must be patient with yourself and even when you have a challenging day, when you might replay some old destructive habits and patterns, that's OK, remember tomorrow is a new day. What is important is that you keep your energy high and don't beat yourself up. Otherwise you are holding on. Accept what has happened and release it. Let it know that it is free to go and thank it for the lessons that you learnt from it.

You see, we're here to learn lessons, and once we get the learning, then we won't be taught that lesson again. There is a great deal of talk about the ego these days and how our ego is our opponent. Something we need to constantly battle against within ourselves. It is talked about like this in many spiritual circles. I have a different understanding to this.

I see the ego as a friend and a training partner for life. I draw an analogy of this from martial arts. Most martial arts focus on fighting an opponent and will have tournaments, competitions and sparring sessions. This can build a competitive ego. The emotions involved are the lower sort, such as pride, determination and even anger. These are useful emotions to utilise at times. No emotion is wrong. They are all there to serve us, and these arts are useful for bringing people who live at lower emotional levels up to new levels.

I teach the art of Budo Taijustsu, where there is no competitiveness whatsoever. It humbles the ego, by letting your training partner apply techniques, then you do the same with them. It is a co-operative flow of energy in accordance with nature's laws. We learn not to resist, because what resists persists. In life our training partner is our ego sharing lessons with us, and if we don't move out of the way of a punch, then we get hit, and we will continue to get hit with the lesson until we take the learning by moving a certain direction. Then we receive a new lesson, maybe in the form of a kick, and then we have to take the learning from that to move to the next level.

As long as we see the ego as our training partner in life, then we will be happy to train with her gratefully, accepting lessons that will move us forward to constantly evolving into the next grandest version of ourselves. So don't resist your ego. Gratefully learn from it. If a person is fat, then they are fat for a reason that will serve them. It is actually a great opportunity for them to transform themselves, as there is really nothing more exciting and fulfilling as transformation, or seeing someone else transform where you have had a part in it.

We are children of God. God didn't deal us a crappy hand of cards so we would have a crappy game. She dealt us that hand, to see how we would play the game. No matter what the hand you have been dealt looks like, be grateful for it, as it is an unbelievable, incomprehensible opportunity to grow, blossom and flourish. We must be so appreciative of the fact that we Get to play the game!

Make each day of your life your masterpiece. Gratefully accept the lessons and take the learnings. Love yourself and find the beauty in everything. What you focus on, you will get more of. You are a being of intricate beauty. You are the most complex, intelligent and powerful system in the known universe. Your potential is infinite. Live boundlessly.

Live like you will die tomorrow, learn like you will live forever
– *Mahatma Gandhi*

These are some of the wisest words ever spoken for life. Do what you love. Do what brings you joy. Do only that. This is an urgent message to you. You have so little time my friend. Live right now. Accept nothing else but who you are at the core of your being. There is no more time for fear or stress or anxiety. You have done enough of that. Take the lesson right now from your ego training partner and step joyously into the flow of life and be surrounded by beauty and love.

You are doing wonderfully by the way, and I have one more tool and technique to share with you in relation to transformation of the mind; and I have saved the best for last. This is the most efficient and effective transformational technique in the world today, and it is called, 'Emotional Freedom Techniques' or EFT for short and it works on ANYTHING.

EFT is a cousin of acupuncture, as it works on stimulating the body's meridian system, releasing blocked energy and balancing the emotions, by harmonising the body's energetic system. You may know a little about EFT as it has grown in popularity recently, and the question I have for you if you do know about it, is are you doing it? Because a lot of people know what to do, but aren't doing what they know. This is all about taking action, and this stuff really works and gets stupendous results, so lets start doing it!

Gary Craig the founder of EFT, termed the phrase, which is the principal that EFT works on *"All negative emotion is a result of a disruption in the body's energy system"*

All negative emotion is a result of a disruption in the body's energy system

What EFT does, is it balances the body's energy system, harmonising any disruptions and ridding the body of all negative emotion. Because our emotions are connected to any blockages we might have, EFT also has a powerful and profound effect on all manner of physical dis-eases.

When we experience a negative emotion, that emotion will actually store itself somewhere in the body, as a physical manifestation. So if you find it difficult to forgive and you have lower back problems then guess where all those unforgiving emotions are hanging out, or if you have a few spare tyres and can't seem to get rid of them its because the anger needs to live somewhere since you haven't freed him yet!

What we are going to focus on here, is how you can do EFT with yourself to assist you in releasing any food cravings and also for negative identity issues.

Play Video 1

In the photograph below you will see the nine points, which you will be tapping on. Follow the numbered sequence while

focusing on the negative issue that you wish to release.
Using four fingers, you will start tapping firmly on the karate chop point, whilst saying a set-up phrase. And you will repeat the phrase three times.

The more emphatically you say it the better. You then go on to the top of the head with four fingers, tapping whilst

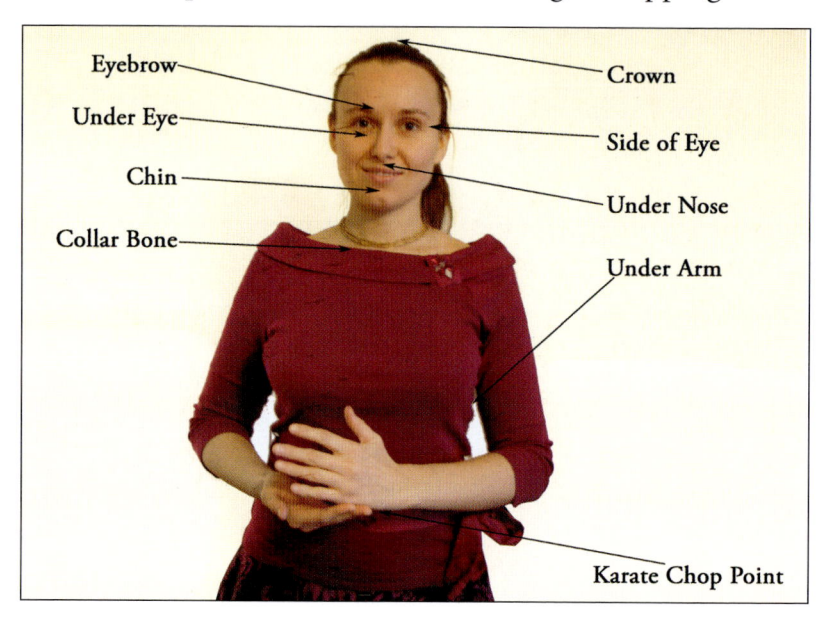

![Tapping points diagram: Eyebrow, Under Eye, Chin, Collar Bone, Crown, Side of Eye, Under Nose, Under Arm, Karate Chop Point]

saying a shortened version, continuing to above the eye with two fingers, then to the side of the eye, then under the eye, then to under the nose, then to the groove between the chin and the lip, then to the collar bone, one inch from the end of the collar bone with four fingers, and then to under the arm with four fingers, just higher than the elbow. Tap five to eight times on each point, focusing on the emotion or issue that you wish to resolve. It's really as simple as that.

Discipline is very important. Some people try it for five minutes and decide that it doesn't work and that is the problem,

all they did was "try". In order to succeed you must do! Do or do not. Try is a human construct.
Persevere with EFT and you will receive the result that you are looking for.

I will give you a personal experience that I had with a client using EFT, that will let you understand how to use it and the huge potential benefits for you in your life. A lady called Jane came to me for coaching. Jane was grossly obese and terribly unhappy. Ashamed was the word she used, which is actually the lowest human emotion. She first told me her "story", and how she had tried everything to lose weight and nothing worked and that she had been fat for so long that it was just impossible for her to lose weight.

We started tapping on the nine points while discussing general issues using the set-up phrases.
"Even though it is impossible for me to lose weight, I deeply and completely accept myself."
Then the shortened version we would say whilst tapping the other eight points was *"impossible for me to lose weight"*

The next one was: *"Even though I am ashamed of myself, I deeply and completely accept myself"*.

Shortened to *"Ashamed of myself."*
Forty-five minutes later we had journeyed deep into her unconscious mind and found ourselves down at the roots. We started getting very specific, and this is critical for effectiveness with EFT, is to get specific. Start off general if you are not sure of the specific issue, and then pathways will be

presented to you that will eventually take you to the root cause.

So with Jane, as we continued tapping, suddenly a flash came to her, of a memory that she had suppressed. The memory was of her at about seven years of age, in which she had returned home after a summer holiday at her grandparents.

Upon opening the front door, her mother peered down at her and said,

"You look a site, look how much weight you've put on"

When this memory came up for Jane, she became very angry and started to cry. I asked her on a scale of zero to ten, (with zero being no negative emotion whatsoever and ten being unbearable agonising pain), how did she feel when she thought of that event. She said it was a ten, and I had a strong feeling that we had arrived at the root of what had manifested as a severe obesity problem.

We started to tap on it.

"Even though my mother told me I looked a site and had put on weight, I deeply and completely accept myself"

Shortened to: *"Mother told me I was a site, and put on weight"* This brought the intensity of the emotion down to a seven.
"Even though she was mean and horrible to me, I deeply and completely accept myself" shortened to: *"Mother mean and horrible to me"*

The intensity came down to five.

"Even though she was probably having a bad day and didn't mean it, I deeply and completely accept myself"

Shortened to *"Having a bad day, and didn't mean it"*
The intensity came down to three.

"Even though I have been holding onto all this pain and weight for so many years, because my mother didn't mean it, I deeply and completely accept myself"

Shortened to *"Holding onto pain and weight, mother didn't mean it."*

This brought it down to zero. So I asked Jane to think of the event and how it made her feel. A bemused look came across her face and she said she was having trouble remembering it, and what she could remember, was like it was something she had seen on TV, and not something that had happened to her.

I then asked her to think of other events that brought up a negative emotion, and she said that there weren't any. What we had done was created a crescendo. We toppled the most significant emotional event and that collapsed the rest.

Jane walked out of my practice that day, not sure of what had happened or how it would change her life.
Almost a year had past, and I was walking down the street, I could see a woman walking in my direction with a smile

on her face, I could see her making eye contact with me, but had no idea who she was. I was about to walk past her, when she stopped in front of me and said "*Hello Matthew.*" Only by her voice and by looking into her eyes, did I realise that it was Jane. Over 30 years of being obese and unhappy had been released. She was totally transformed. She was slim. She had released over 80 pounds of unforgiving hurt and anger. There was a sparkle in her eye, a spring in her step and forgiveness in her heart.

If there is some weight that you need to release, what I recommend is, if it is forty pounds or whatever it is, put the equivalent in a bag and carry it everywhere you go for the next 24 hours, even to the bathroom. Feel how it limits your day and lowers your standard of living and well-being. This will give you an idea of the contrast, as this is utilising the law of contrast. I really recommend you don't just think about it, actually do it, and it will be an uncomfortable 24 hours, and what you will get at the end of it, is a huge relief and then you will have the contrast, so you can feel what it will be like when you release the forty pounds around your waist. You see if you put a frog into boiling water, it will jump out, but if you put a frog into cold water and gently heat it up, the frog will boil to death. Side-note: Please don't test this!

Most people put on weight and get out of shape over time, so they don't realise the detrimental effect it is having on them, (*unfortunately for most*) until it is too late.
So now you have the basics of EFT, start applying it and make it a habit.

I will now share with you again the profoundly powerful mantra that is in strict accordance with the truth. Go through the EFT tapping sequence whilst saying it. Go through it three times tapping on all nine points whilst saying:

I am whole, perfect, strong, powerful, loving, harmonious and happy

I recommend that you do this everyday. First thing in the morning is a good time!

Do you see what we are doing here? We are ridding the mind of all negative emotions, releasing patterns that no longer serve us. This is total purification of the mind, of any and all mistaken identities, because that was the problem. It was a mistaken identity. You had simply forgotten who you are at your core. You have now realised that you are not fat, and that there is nothing wrong with you. You are actually whole, you are perfect, you are strong, you are powerful, you are loving, you are harmonious, and yes you are happy my friend. This is true self realisation.

These are not things you must find outside of yourself; they are all there in you already. Realise them by surrendering to yourself. Let go of any resistance, breathing deeply and relaxing your body helps. Allow your true self to emerge. You don't need to make anything happen. Just as the water in the river runs down the mountainside, it allows nature to take its course. When the water flows into the rock, it does not stop and procrastinate in which direction it should be flowing. It simply trusts that the universal nature knows where it is going and it follows, flowing around the rock making its way down towards the sea with great ease; accepting it's true nature, because it is water that makes up the river, and that is what the river does.

My friend you too are water, studies now suggest that we are made up of 98% water. Whatever you do, do not stagnate, be like water my friend, because you are, and keep on flowing.

This now brings us to the completion of part one. Although this is not the end of your mind training, in-fact this is just the beginning; now that you have the tools and techniques, and I envisage that you have already made some huge shifts in your thinking, making new distinctions, new learning's and discoveries of who you really are and what you are capable of. Which will in turn impact your life, making possible, what you once thought impossible.

If for whatever reason you did not complete the exercises in part one, now is the time to do them before you move to reading part two. Even if you only left out one exercise, do it…. because the reason for not doing them is fear and we really do not want to make decisions out of fear. Procrastination of "I will do it later" or rationalisation of "I don't need to do it" even if you are being an exemplary student and you completed all exercises, I invite you to read part one again anyway, as there is a great deal in it, and a second reading will bring up new distinctions for you.

This time there will also be something different. Because now you know, understand and can apply EFT, what you will do, is at the end of each page, do a quick round of EFT on whatever comes up at the time. If you are feeling great, then tap on that. If you come to an exercise that you haven't already completed and you don't wish to do it, tap on that and feel the negative emotion and any association dissolve away.

You see there is no failure as long as you take the action and keep going no matter what. In this case, failure is quitting, and the truth is, that you cannot quit. This is your life. Every second that goes by, you have less time here. You cannot buy this day back with the entire fortune of Bill Gates. You must take action and you must act in spite of fear. Laugh and be joyous as this is your true nature. I dare you to smile right now. Ha ha, got ya. You are truly magnificent!

Part 2 - Nutrition

"Nothing tastes as good as fit, healthy and vital feels"
– Anthony Robbins

Food, Nutrition and liquid. The stuff that fuels your body. I am going to start this with the most important and profound statement there is regarding health, nutrition and weight release. It's not what you eat that makes the biggest difference, it's how you eat it.

It's not what you eat that makes the biggest difference, it's how your eat it

What do I mean by this? Well you could eat the healthiest, organic, nutritious food, but if you are swallowing it, before you get a chance to taste it, let alone chew it, you are doing your body harm. Food gets clogged in your stomach and your intestines, and your internal organs have to work double shifts to try and break that food down, putting a great deal of stress and strain on the body. If you eat when you are stressed, again it doesn't matter how healthy and nutritious that food is, it turns to poison as it enters your digestive system, because it comes into energetic resonance with how you are feeling emotionally.

If you eat while you have your mind on other things, like maybe watching the TV or reading, or talking or thinking about your day at work, this also has a detrimental effect on the body.

Another reason we must slow down our eating is so that we know when we have had enough. If we gulp our food down in ten minutes, we will quite often go for a second helping, because we don't feel full or satisfied. Then after we have finished the second helping, we feel over full or uncomfortably full and we have also expanded or stretched our stomach, so then the next time we eat, we can actually fit more food in and the process continues. If we had waited for 15 minutes after completing our first meal, we would have received a message from our digestive system telling us, that we have had enough, and we would then feel satisfied. Even better than that, eat the meal slower; fully masticating, which will take us thirty minutes to eat. Then by the time we finish, we will know that we have had enough.

Is the statement starting to make sense? It's not what you eat that determines your health and waistline; it's how you eat it. Over 95% of fat people eat too fast. And they don't eat too fast because they are fat, they are fat because they eat too fast. Slow the feck down! I say this to interrupt any passive readers, because this is of vital importance that you start creating correct eating habits before you start concerning yourself with what you put in your mouth. So although everything in this book is mucho important, I am writing in order of importance, from the inside out, because once you change things in your inner environment, your outer environment starts to naturally correspond and resonate with your inner environment.

Chew, chew, chew, your food

Each mouthful fifty times. Yes fifty times. Your food must turn into liquid before you swallow it. Your mouth is where food is predigested, and by chewing it, you send a message to your stomach, to prepare for it, so your stomach prepares for the food by creating the correct amount of stomach acid to further break down and digest it, so it can then enter the intestines, for absorption into the body as nutrients.

Drink your solids and chew your liquids

This is a quote from the Grandfather of the natural health movement in the USA. Paul Bragg lived until he was ninety-seven years young and died as a result of a surfing accident. Most people are long gone before they reach this age, and those that aren't are usually unable to leave the house, or nursing home and are merely surviving. Paul Bragg was surfing the waves, when he decided it was time to depart, and he lived by these principals.

Do you agree that you are getting a great deal more, than you bargained for in this book? Not only are you going to be thin, look great and feel great. You will also have a greater possibility for longevity. Growing old with passion and energy.

So when would it now be a good time to start incorporating some of these habits? That's right...NOW!

From now on, when you eat anything, be like a Zen monk, being very conscious of what you are putting in your mouth and why! Remember food isn't something we should do to get feelings from. Food is fuel, it is nourishment, it is energy and it is nutrition. As you eat each mouthful, be in the present. Make eating like your meditation. Counting each mouthful fifty chews before swallowing.

After doing this consistently for a month or two, it will then become a habit, and counting will no longer be necessary as you will naturally chew your food until it becomes liquid, and you will naturally then swallow it without gulping.

By doing this you are giving your internal organs a huge gift, as in the past, they have been working so hard and are really in need of a rest. It also takes a massive amount of energy for your digestive system to break down food that hasn't been chewed thoroughly, and that is why most people become tired after a meal, because all the body's energy has gone to the digestive system. When your meal is chewed thoroughly this will not happen. Food is fuel, and food is energy. It is not supposed to zonk us out!

If you do what we have talked about up until now, without even changing your diet or incorporating any sort of exercise plan, you will experience massive shifts and a positive transformation of yourself. One last time.... "It's not what you eat that makes the biggest difference, it is how you eat it."

Now, what I'm going to share with you is nutritionally a major key to releasing unwanted weight. We have an acid-alkaline balance in our bodies. Our blood is slightly alkaline, and holds at a steady 7.365 on the pH scale. If this varies by only a few points we can become ill and die. This is similar to our body temperature, which is a steady 37.5 degrees Celsius or 98.6 degrees Fahrenheit. If this varies by a few degrees we can become sick and die.

So our bodies are slightly alkaline and will do anything to keep it that way. Otherwise we wouldn't survive. The problem is, that in today's society people live an acid lifestyle!

What do I mean by that. Well, we eat acidic foods, drink acidic drinks, feel acidic emotions, do acidic activities breathe in acidic air in an acidic way...not to mention the acidic affect from mobile phones, computers and all the other electromagnetic chaos going on all around us. Which also compromises our inner terrain and causes a build up of acid.

And you wonder what does all this have to do with you releasing 25 pounds of excess weight? As a protection mechanism, our body stores acid in its fat stores to protect the internal organs, (which keeps the body alive) from becoming over acid. Do you get what I am saying here?

People aren't over weight, they are over acid
– Dr Robert Young

People aren't over weight they are over acid, which shows up as being over weight. We must alkalise our bodies, which will energise us. This is what will flush out the excess acid, and guess what? We have already been doing it throughout this book, by raising our emotional vibration, which is actually the most important factor in alkalising our bodies.

To give you an example, years ago I used to promote alkalising products, which were very potent and produced great results. One of my clients came to me and said that the product he was using wasn't working, and all they made him do was feel sick. I asked him about his life and what was going on, and he proceeded to tell me that he was constantly stressed about everything. His kids stressed him, his wife stressed him, his business stressed him and world events stressed him. Even in his sleep he was stressed and would wake up in a cold sweat regularly.

I explained to him that the product was very potent and effective and it was his emotions that were overriding its effectiveness. The sick feeling he was having, was the product giving him a cleansing crisis, which is where it dumps out a lot of toxins and acid in one go, which first has to travel from the fat stores and through the body for release. What he was doing was poring a constant stream of acid into his body from his mind. So, no matter how much alkaline juice he put into his body, it was fighting a losing battle.

Do you appreciate why we are only getting into the nutrition side of things now? And by the way, just to put your mind at rest, I am not going to ask you to give up or cut out anything from your nutritional plan, although there are a few food additives to be aware of. What will naturally happen as you start to add more alkaline food and drinks, is that you will naturally not crave acidic foods or drinks so much, and you will gravitate to food and drink that is of an alkaline nature.

"You are what you eat" became a very popular saying a few years ago, that was tossed about in the diet and nutrition industry. Well we have already discovered that it is not what you eat...yes you got it, it's HOW you eat it.

There is another vitally important part to add to the puzzle, because really that's what it is, it's a puzzle. People are fat because they are puzzled. They have been told all these different things from the so-called health experts. "Diet this" and "Low fat that". Have you ever noticed that when you are in your local food outlet that the people who buy the "Diet this and low fat that" are mostly fat! And the people who don't aren't! This is because that crap doesn't work. The food industry doesn't want people to be thin; otherwise people wouldn't eat so much and the food industries profits would go down. They want to fatten people up so they buy more food, and in turn they can fatten their wallets. The "low this" and "diet that" are loaded with chemicals that produce food cravings in the body.

Ok, so lets get forward on track. The second most important food principal is:

It's not what you eat, it's when you eat it

If you eat before you go to bed, then that food is not getting burned off and is going straight to your fat stores whilst you sleep. You are also not getting a proper night's sleep because your internal organs are working throughout the night whilst you sleep. So do you ever wonder why you find it hard to get out of bed in the morning, and that you regularly feel tired throughout the day. Hmm, something to think about!

Do not eat anything at least three hours before you go to bed

So do not eat anything at least three hours before you go to bed. And if you feel any hunger pangs or cravings, fill yourself a glass of water and drink as much as you need until they subside. I recommend that the first thing you drink in the morning is a large glass of slightly warmed water with half a lemon squeezed into it. Lemons although they are a citric acid, convert to alkaline when in the body. They are extremely good for you, a great kidney cleanser and overall cleanser of the body, loaded with vitamin C! I would generally squeeze half a lemon into my water a few times a day.

Water is the most important substance we put into our bodies and we really can't get enough of it. Drink it regularly, as often our thirst signals are confused and we believe we are hungry and reach for some food, when really we are thirsty. I have heard it said by so called "health experts" that we should only drink when we are thirsty, which is garbage! As a person ages, the senses on their tongue that tell them when they are thirsty become less effective and again can also be confused for being hungry.

Drink good water, have a water filter installed, it is one of the best investments you will ever make. Drink at the very least two litres of water per day. And contrary to popular belief, more water does not add to water retention, it actually reverses it, as water retention is the body's survival device because it is not getting enough water, so it holds onto it.

Once the body knows that it is receiving water regularly, then it will let go of water retention. Water will also flush out toxins including the acid waste that is in the fat stores. Here are a few signals to let you know if you are dehydrated.

1. **Yellow urine** – It should be clear!
2. **Constipation** – Our body needs fluids for bowel movements!
3. **Lethargy and feeling tired** – water is an energiser!
4. **Darkness around the eyes** is a toxic build-up that can be flushed away with water!
5. **Premature wrinkles on skin** – water moisturises the skin and helps keep elasticity! If you experience any of these five, then the chances are you are severely dehydrated.

Right now, I would invite you to drink one pint of water, which is over half a litre. If you have a lemon there then squeeze some in! Take note of how you feel beforehand, even look in the mirror to see how you look. Now how do you look and feel after that? Clearer, more energised is the usual response from just one pint of water and lemon.

Do you like to drink tea? Green Tea is the number one tea you could possibly drink. In Japan, when you walk into any restaurant, you traditionally have a cup of Green Tea placed in front of you. A fat Japanese person is a very rare sight, unless you go to watch the sumo wrestling and those guys work very hard to get as big as they are.

Green Tea can have an acquired taste, so start off having it weak and you will soon love it. And by the way, I am not saying that the majority or Japanese are thin because they drink green tea, what I am saying is that it is a large contributor as it speeds up the metabolism, helps burn fat, and it is also full of health giving properties, including anti-oxidants.

I am now going to make another profound statement.

Its not what you eat, it's what you excrete!

You see there is a problem in the world, and it is that people are full of shit! Literally. We need to flush it out of our bodies daily. When John Wayne died, the autopsy revealed that his colon weighed 82 pounds!! If you were given a bag with eighty two pounds of crap in it to carry around everywhere you went, you wouldn't be long getting rid of it. Because it is hidden inside people, they don't realise it's there, and so don't do anything about it.

Even thin people are full of it! I had a colonic irrigation when I was four percent body fat and had been cleansing on Juices and water for five days with no solid food whatsoever. You would think that there would be nothing left in me, but the colonic removed about six pounds of crap from my intestines, and I am sure that there was more there if I would have had further colonic's.

Colonic's are great and I highly recommend them. If you are really serious about your health and achieving your ideal weight, book a series of colonic's right now. Grab the yellow pages, or go on-line, there is somewhere near you that does them and it doesn't hurt. It is clean and you will feel amazing afterwards. Go ahead, do it right now. You see it is in our intestines that most of the nutrition is absorbed into our blood stream and transported to the cells all around our body.

If our intestines are full of crap, then it doesn't matter how nutritious the food is that we are eating, it gets absorbed into the crap, instead of into our blood. If the thought of going for a colonic is too much right now, then there are colon cleanses that we can ingest in capsule form and powders that can be mixed with water and drank.

There are two great value drinks that I recommend for cleansing the bowels and intestines. I drink both daily. The first is home made Kombucha Tea, which is many times more powerful than the packaged versions you can buy in the shops, and although it is made using sugar, most of the sugar is absorbed into the Kombucha Culture in the fermentation process and the rest is transmuted and is good for you. Kombucha is very effective in supporting weight release, as it is a powerful detoxifier. It speeds up the metabolism and acts like an internal poultice pulling all the crap out of the body. I would go as far as to say that Kombucha is a miracle.

Drink three glasses of it a day. Purchase your home kit, and start brewing immediately.

Order at **www.bethinfeelgreat.net**

The second is Molasses, which is really overlooked. It is inexpensive, great value and can be purchased from any health food store. It is packed full of the Earth's minerals, B-Vitamins and Iron. Start off by taking a teaspoon in a mug with a little cold water, and then pour in boiling water stir and drink. As your taste buds become more accustomed to it, you can increase it to a tablespoon. Drink up to three mugs of it per day. After your glass of Kombucha is a good time, as the two together, make for an amazing combination to cleanse the bowels adding much needed nutrients to the body.

If you do not immediately enjoy the taste when you have your first glass of Kombucha or mug of Molasses, that's fine. You can start off by adding a little apple juice to the Kombucha and with the molasses just take less and build it up, because let me ask you a question! When you first started drinking beer or wine, did you like it immediately? More often than not, the answer is no, of course not. Most people start by drinking Shandy's and light wines and then acquire the taste. This can be a similar experience, and remember that Kombucha and molasses are much, much better for you than beer or wine! And they will help your body transform and become more alkaline. It is a great thing when your body becomes alkaline because then your taste buds tune to alkaline foods and drinks and you stop craving acidic foods.

So, if you have been waiting for me to tell you what you need to 'cut out', think again! Focus on the good stuff, put as much of it into your body as possible, and the not so good stuff will disappear from your life. Where focus goes, energy flows! Focus on the good stuff!

This is a profoundly simple and effective way to live a successful life.... Focus on the good stuff.

Vegetables are the number one food group that you must be eating. The best way to get vegetables into your body is through juicing. Have you bought that Juicer yet that we talked about earlier in the book? You can buy whole fruit juicers, which can juice whole apples without cutting them up. Which is very convenient. At least get a mid-range juicer, as you will pay more in time and juice loss, by buying a cheap one.

Make juicing a part of your daily life! Do not have it in a cupboard, have it on display between your toaster and kettle and use it every day. There is no better way of getting nutrients into your body than juicing, and if you are still beating the drum of *But I want to lose weight, who cares about these nutrients"* I will let you in on a little secret.

When the body is nutrient deficient, the signals show up as *"I am hungry"*.. You are not hungry! You are dehydrated and lacking in nutrition.

You are not hungry! You are dehydrated and lacking in nutrition.

In fact, drink a pint of water right now, and squeeze half a lemon into it while you are at it. I don't care if you just had one ten minutes ago, have another, because really how many alcoholic drinks might you drink on a night out. Now sit up in your chair and take a few deep diaphramic breaths, feeling great!

Most people when they start juicing mainly juice fruits. I say, eat your fruits and juice your vegetables.

Eat your fruits and juice your vegetables.

Use carrots as your sweetener and start off with two thirds carrot juice and one third green juice, which could be Cucumber, Celery, Broccoli, Cabbage, Spinach or a mixture of these which are all highly alkaline.

Through time you can slowly switch to two-thirds green juice, and one third carrot. An alternative to carrot is apple for juice drinks, and apples are the only fruit that I would advise to mix with vegetables for juice drinks. As a treat what is really great is four apples, one pineapple, and half a lemon all juiced together.

If you have a high performance juicer, then you can put the pineapple in with the skin, which is really good for you. Doing this with other juicers will blunt the blades. If you are using organic lemons then juice the skin as well, as this is also really good for you. Non-organic lemons, will have been sprayed with chemicals, and therefore should be peeled.

Play Video 2

While we are on the subject of Organic, an organic tomato has roughly 2000 times more Iron in it than a non-organic tomato. Organic food is more expensive, and you are really getting your money's worth. So when you have the choice, buy it!

The optimum time to drink veggie-juice drinks is on an empty stomach, so first thing in the morning and before meals is best. If you are drinking them after you have eaten, then they are losing some of the effect, by being absorbed into the food and they can produce an unhealthy reaction with certain foods.

Trophology – This is the science of food combining. The reason we would combine some foods and not others is because some foods do not react well together while going through the digestive process. If you don't eat meat or fish, then you do not need to be too concerned with food combining. It is mixing meat with carbohydrates, such as pasta, Potatoes, Bread or Rice that is the main problem.

A family member of mine shed over 60 pounds in three months, by simply eating his carbohydrates at lunch and his proteins at dinner. He didn't change what he ate, he only changed when he ate it. So as far as Trophology goes, my main recommendations are; if you eat meat and fish then only eat it in the evening, with salad and vegetables, without any carbohydrates. As meat is difficult for the body to digest, I would also recommend not drinking anything with your meal and for at least one hour after finishing. Otherwise you are diluting the stomach acids, which help break the meat down.

Most fruit should be eaten on an empty stomach, especially oranges as they react with everything. Can you see that I am making it really simple? Whole books have been written on Trophology and other things that I have shared with you in these pages. I am keeping it simple so that you get it and apply it.

Decide now, that for the next twenty-four hours, you will combine your food correctly.

Eat a salad with every meal. This will alkalise any acidity that is in the rest of your meal. It will give your body a lot of the nutrients and enzymes that it needs, as most nutrients are killed off in the cooking process, and it acts as a filler so you don't eat as much.

So how much of this are you highlighting and taking notes on? And how much are you going to make part of your daily routine? Do all of it, and you will be transformed. Make that decision **NOW** and you are transformed!
Here follows a small list of foods for you to introduce into your nutritional plan.

> **1. Sprouted wheat bread** – I would eat this instead of other breads. Real sprouted wheat bread is stodgy.
> **2. Quinoa** – As I don't eat meat, this gives me my essential amino acids.

3. Brown Rice – I would eat this instead of Pasta.

4. Homous and Tahini – Both go great on sprouted wheat bread, and act as a great dip for raw vegetables!

5. Celtic Ocean Sea Salt – Instead of other salts. It is full of minerals.

6. Avocados – These are just so good for you and go great on sprouted wheat bread.

Add these to your shopping list now. You should be able to purchase them from your nearest health food store.

Make it fun and start experimenting. Maybe you already eat some of them and that's great. Start eating really nourishing foods and your body will love you for it!

As you can see the principals and plan in this book is not to deprive you of anything, it is to add to your palette, add to your life and add to your experience of becoming more of who you are.

Please reread this, take notes. Highlight the main principals and start today to transform yourself through your eating and drinking habits.

What follows is a seven day nutritional plan, which can act as a guideline for you and a great starting point.

Day One

Morning	Glass of warm water with lemon, one pint of vegetable juice (cucumber, celery, carrots.)
Mid-morning	One banana, glass of water and lemon, green tea.
Lunch	Water and lemon, mixed salad, sprouted wheat bread with homous and avocado, glass of kombucha
Evening	Kombucha, water and lemon, molasses, mixed salad, vegetable stir fry with brown rice.
Late Evening	Kombucha, green tea, water and lemon.

Day Two

Morning	Warm water with lemon. 1 pint of juice (broccoli, spinach & apples) ***Note:** Use 1 full broccoli, cut the heads off and keep for dinner.*
Mid-morning	Avocado, green tea
Afternoon	Water & lemon, salad, sprouted wheat bread, homous & sliced tomato, kombucha
Evening	Kombucha, molasses, green tea, salad, quinoa with brown rice, stir fry (broccoli, mushrooms, onions).
Late Evening	Kombucha, Green Tea, Water & Lemon.

Day Three

Morning	Glass of warm water with lemon, one pint of vegetable juice (cucumber, cabbage, carrot).
Mid-morning	Mixture of dried fruit, nuts and seeds, and green tea.
Lunch	Water and lemon, mixed salad, sprouted wheat bread with tahini and avocado, glass of kombucha.
Evening	Kombucha, molasses, green tea, mixed salad, home made vegetable soup.
Late Evening	Kombucha, green tea, water and lemon.

Day Four

Morning	Glass of warm water with lemon, one pint of vegetable juice (celery, spinach and apple)
Mid-morning	Banana and green tea
Lunch	Water and lemon, mixed salad, quinoa with homous, green tea.
Evening	Kombucha, molasses, green tea mixed salad, roasted potatoes and vegetables.
Late Evening	Kombucha, green tea, water and lemon.

Day Five

Morning	Glass of warm water with lemon, one pint of vegetable juice (celery, broccoli and carrot).
Mid-morning	Avocado, and green tea.
Lunch	Water and lemon, mixed salad, sprouted wheat bread with sun dried tomatoes, homous, glass of kombucha.
Evening	Kombucha, molasses, green tea, mixed salad, mashed potatoes mixed with onions, cabbage, sweet corn and broccoli.
Late Evening	Kombucha, green tea, water and lemon.

Day Six

Morning	Glass of warm water with lemon, one pint of vegetable juice (cucumber, celery and apple).
Mid-morning	Flapjack, and green tea.
Lunch	Water and lemon, mixed salad, sprouted wheat bread with tahini, avocado and tomato, glass of kombucha.
Evening	Kombucha, molasses, green tea, mixed salad, vegetable curry and brown rice.
Late Evening	Kombucha, green tea, water and lemon.

Day Seven

Morning	Glass of warm water with lemon, one glass of juice (pineapple, lemon and apple). Porridge made with water, mix in pumpkin seeds, sesame seeds, raw almonds and maple syrup.
Mid-morning	Green tea
Lunch	Water and lemon, mixed salad with meal of your choice and dessert, kombucha.
Evening	Kombucha, molasses, green tea, mixed salad, Home made tomato soup with brown rice.
Late Evening	Kombucha, green tea, water and lemon.

With the salads be adventurous. Mix in a boiled egg (Free Range and Organic), bell peppers, broccoli, spinach, carrots (finely chopped or shredded), some spring onions.

Everything should be made as simple as possible, but not simpler
– Albert Einstein

You can see that I have kept the nutritional plan simple. This is by design. Because if I gave you an executive chef style menu, it would all look like too much hassle and create overwhelm and you probably wouldn't do any of it. I have given you a little variety and again not too much, because we really don't need that much variety in our food.

It is only in recent years that people have started eating a very varied diet, because food gets shipped to us from all over the world and companies are competing with each other by supplying as many different foods and drinks as possible. The generations before us really only ate what was locally produced, which created very little variety. We don't need much variety. It is an unnecessary luxury!

Make sure that the food you eat is fresh, organic when possible and FREE of chemicals; *including preservatives, additives, flavourings, especially Monosodium Glutamate, Aspartame, Hydrogenated Vegetable Oil - Trans Fats.* **This is the bad stuff!** Avoid it at all costs.

Just keep putting the good stuff in!

Educate yourself and take responsibility for your health. Don't take my word for it either. Google anything that you are not sure of or want to know more about. Inevitably you can find both positive and negative information about most things on this planet, so do your own research and make your own informed decisions!

For the finale of the second part of this book, I will leave you with a fool proof method of testing if something is good for you, or bad for you,. Or if something is truthful or false.
You can do this using Kinesiology, or what is commonly know as muscle testing. Test this out with a willing person. You will hold your right arm out to the side horizontally and the other person will place two fingers on your wrist, while facing you. They will ask you the question "Is your name...

(then they will say your real name)
You answer "Yes"

They say "Resist", while they push down on your arm. You will be strong and your arm will put up a lot of resistance.

They will then ask you the same question again, this time inserting a different name. Even though this is not your name, you answer "yes".

They say "resist" and push down on your arm, this time because you have lied, it will have weakened your body and you will not be able to put up much resistance and your arm will easily be pushed down.

This technique can be used on pretty much anything, because your body does not lie, it knows!

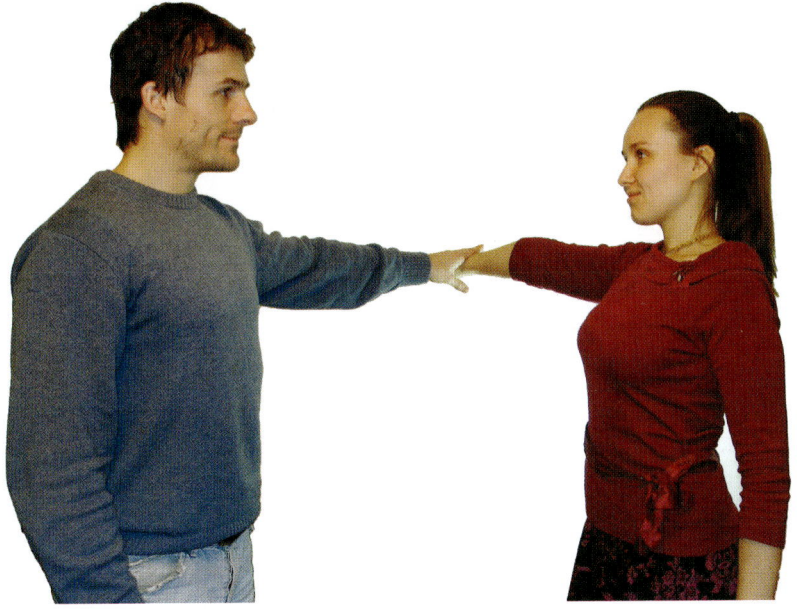

Use muscle testing when you are doing your shopping. Any item you pick up, to know whether it will be good for you or not, simply hold it in your left hand against your solar plexus (stomach) and get the person with you to ask if it is good for you. If you test weak then it is not.

You can also do this test when you are by yourself. Press the tip of your ring finger on your left hand against the tip of your thumb creating pressure. Now take your index finger on your other hand, and quickly slide your index finger between your thumb and ring finger. If your finger and thumb separate and your index finger passes through that means you have tested weak. If your finger and thumb stay together, that means you have tested strong. Like most things, doing this accurately takes practice. This is a gem and a great resource to have at your disposal.

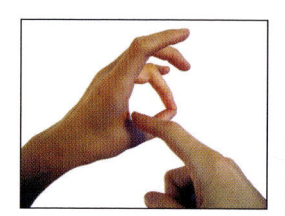

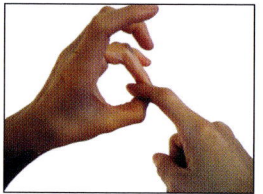

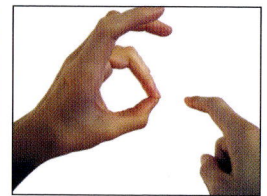

I have used muscle testing a number of times with pregnant women, who want to know the sex of their child. The hospital in my home town refuses to tell the expecting mothers the sex of their baby, as they had a case in the past were they got it wrong and the parents sued. The hospital should have used muscle testing to find out, because I haven't got it wrong yet. Although it wasn't actually me getting it right, it was just their body telling me. This is because the body knows the right answer every time.

Again you don't have to take my word for it if anything in this book is good for you or works. Muscle test it. Even muscle test the book. Hold it against your body and see if you test strong. If for whatever reason you don't, send it back to me and I will give you a refund.

This is how certain I am about the contents of this book and the results that you will achieve by putting what is in these pages into practice. It's really not that hard either. It is simply creating some new habits that will become second nature and will totally transform your life. Enjoy the process, have fun, be proactive and throw all and any caution to the wind as you enter the third part.

Part 3 - Exercise

"No citizen has the right to be an amateur in the matter of physical training. What a disgrace it is for a man to grow old without ever seeing the beauty and strength of which his body is capable."

– Socrates

Movement, motion, exercise. – The stuff that we are made for! Have you ever examined your body? I mean really looked at it. Your joints, tendons, muscles, the mechanics of the whole physical system. Wow, it is totally amazing and I am really feeling the wow factor and how amazing it is, just by thinking about it right now. Take a few minutes now to really study the magnificence of your physical self.

We were born to move! Some people take it to the extreme, such as Olympic gymnasts who posses extraordinary ability in the movement of their bodies. They have pushed the limits of what the human body is capable of.

Some people have gone to the other extreme, and our society supports that. Most people don't really move very much these days. Most people either sit or stand at work. They have mechanical transport so they don't have to walk anywhere. It takes them from their home to work or anywhere else they want to go. When they are at home they spend the majority or the time laying back watching the box, with only a small movement of a finger to change channel. Whilst out and about, stairs have become a thing of the past. With elevators and escalators everywhere. Automatic cars, power steering and cruise control make driving almost passive. Can you remember the days before power steering? Driving was a real workout!

This is most peoples lifestyle and unless you take responsibility for your own movement and play a sport or join a health club, (and actually go) or take part in some sort of physical exercise, your body will start to rapidly deteriorate as there are no demands being put on it.

You must exercise for at least 30 minutes a day, six days a week.

You must exercise for at least 30 minutes a day, six days a week and that is it. If you are thinking that *"I don't have 30 minutes a day"* Let me ask you a question... How much TV do you watch every day? Or if it's work that takes up your time, then exercise for 30 minutes a day and you will be around a lot longer so you will be able to work more and watch more TV, if that's what you're into that is.
Even 30 minutes less sleep per night would be inconceivably more beneficial than not exercising for at least 30 minutes per day. Ok, have we blown all the excuses out of the water yet? Oh wait, there is one more that really blows my

mind, the illogicity of it is just insane! And it is..Wait for it...
"Before I start exercising, I have to get fit first"

I have heard this so many times; I then explain to the person that it is the exercise that gets them fit. It is going to the class that gets them in shape. It is playing the sport that helps them release weight.

Now, I am glad that you don't fit into any of the above, and that you are way past any ridiculous excuses, and that's great!

Right now, write down that you commit to 30 minutes of exercise 6 days a week. You owe this to yourself. Do it now!

_____
_____
_____
_____
_____

Now write down your compelling reason why you commit to this, because remember, your why is your driving force.

_____
_____
_____
_____
_____
_____
_____

The number one time you could possibly exercise is first thing in the morning before you have eaten anything. This is because you will be drawing all your energy from your fat stores and not from the food that you have just eaten. The last time you will have eaten will have been about 12 hours previous. So you wanna see fat burn? This is how you do it baby!

The programme that I am setting out for you here is six days per week, with three days of walking or running depending on what your body will permit at this time. Walking at a brisk pace over hilly terrain is ideal, although anything is infinitely better than nothing.

Work to become a nose breather even while exercising. This is not easy so you can build up slowly. It is my experience that mouth breathers tend to have the poorest health and highest levels of stress. The native American Indians would train their children to only breathe through their nose and Genghis Khan would give his children a mouth full of water and send them for a run up the mountain and back. He would check that they still had the water in their mouth upon their return.

You will walk, jog or run on a Tuesday, Thursday and Saturday. The first ten minutes you will go through your EFT tapping sequence, tapping the nine points and focusing on any fears that might arise, any worries, anything disempowering and any obstacles you have put in your way. Doing this will dissolve any and all negative emotion.

The second ten minutes, you will focus on everything that you are grateful for in your life, and if you are not in a crowded park you can say them out loud emphatically with a big smile on your face. Well, you can actually do this in a crowded park. Start a new trend, and if anyone asks you what you are doing, tell them to buy this book and it will transform their life!

And the final ten minutes you will spend visualising your identity and how your life looks now you are that person. I say it like this, because in order for you to have everything in your life that you want, you must be that person to attract those things. For instance if you want to be a famous celebrity in the entertainment industry, just by visualising yourself being that is not enough. There is an important piece of the puzzle, which I believe is the missing link to visualisation and peoples understanding of the law of attraction.

To be a famous celebrity you must first be confident, be disciplined, be a risk taker, be courageous, and you must be unreasonable. You see, reasonable people live reasonably good lives. Unreasonable people, rise to great heights, because they don't listen to the reasonable people telling them to be reasonable. Is this making sense? Read it a few times, so that you really feel what I am saying rather than just getting it on an intellectual level. So when doing your visualisation, see the person that you are in your heart and soul, before the conditioning of life set in. When you are that person, then the universe will correspond to the vibration your heart is transmitting, by tuning your life to the frequency of your heart. Realisation of your true self is the key.

When you start walking, jogging or running, you will find that thirty minutes won't be enough, and you'll want to increase your distance. This will happen naturally, which is great. So that is the three days of the week taken care of. And now for the Monday, Wednesday and Friday, you will be doing The Complete Physical Conditioning System. This is a system of exercise that I created, which encompasses dynamic yoga postures, ancient Taoist movements and exercises, and western resistance training to offer you a lifelong, safe and effective system of training. Each session takes approximately 30 minutes and can be done at home.

I developed this after years of training and practising the various disciplines, and have taken the best from each and integrated them into an intense 30 minute workout. Of course this can be taken at your own pace and you can build up as you go along.

The reason I did this, is because I focused on western style exercise for many years and found that it was incomplete! I would pick up injuries and even though I was strong and powerful on the outside, and I physically looked in good shape, on the inside I was weak, my health wasn't that great, and my flexibility suffered. I then put all my focus into eastern disciplines, becoming more flexible, relieving my injuries, developing more internal energy and again I felt incomplete. By my standards I was skinny, not as happy with my appearance, and I didn't feel that raw strength and power that I used to have. To do a regular routine in the gym, takes about one and a half hours. A yoga class lasts about one and a half hours as well. I also did some training with some

Korean Taoist Masters, which I felt was incredibly beneficial. To do all this in one day would take about four hours, so it was out of my frustration of wanting to do it all, that led me to drawing the best from each, and condensing it into what I believe is the most effective and complete 30 minute training routine available today!

There are two routines that I will share with you here. Both are different and equally as powerful. If you just do one routine for the rest of your life, that would be fantastic, the benefits you would receive are immeasurable. Do both routines, maybe one for six months and then move to the other and you can swap around every few months; this will bring you to another level again of total well-being!

COMPLETE PHYSICAL CONDITIONING SYSTEM (CPCS)
Routine One

Apparatus Needed: Rebounder, Swiss Ball

Rebounders have been used for years by NASA as an integral part of their astronauts training regime. They are very low impact and they energise every cell in your body. They promote circulation, especially of the lymphatic system helping to flush toxins out of the body and much more.

Swiss balls are very effective at building your core stabiliser muscles. They improve balance and concentration. A workout using the swiss ball burns up a lot of energy as so much of the focus is on keeping yourself stable throughout the exercise. In essence you will work muscles you did not know you had.

First 5 minutes of routine on rebounder.

The following pictures show ten different movements on the rebounder with each set of motions taking 30 seconds and then moving onto the next totalling five minutes.

THE REBOUNDER

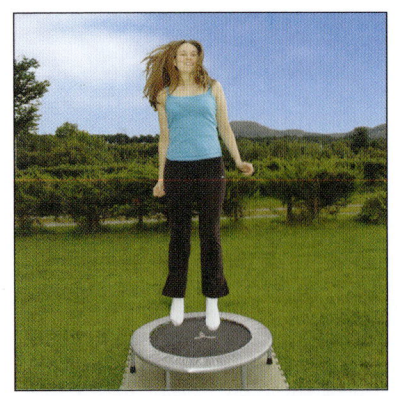

Bouncing sraight up and down

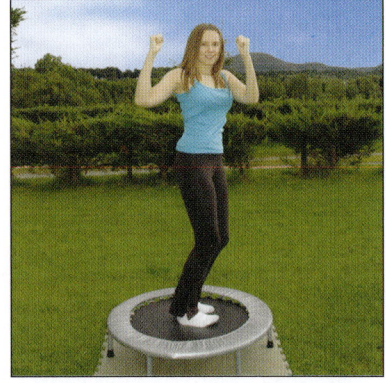

Bouncing whilst twisting hips one way and shoulders the other way.

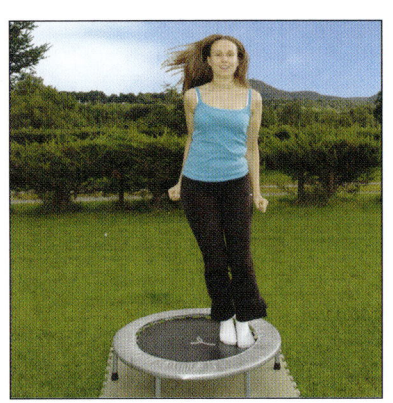

Skiing side to side.

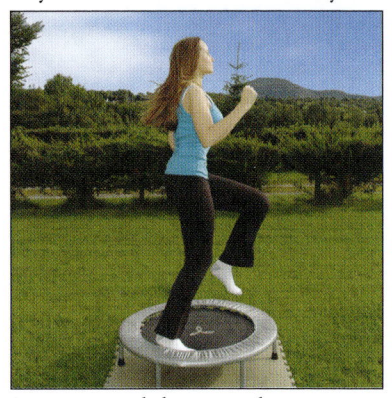

Running with knees in the air.

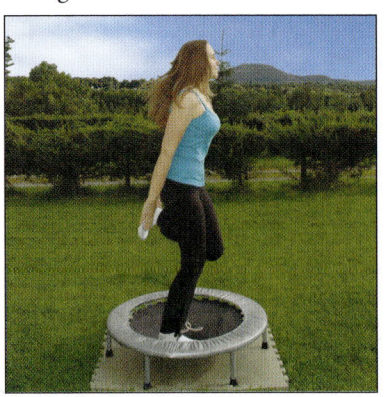

Running with heals up

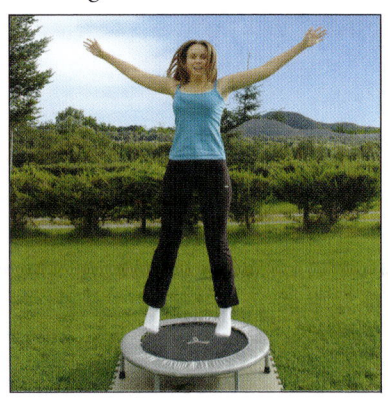

Jumping Jacks

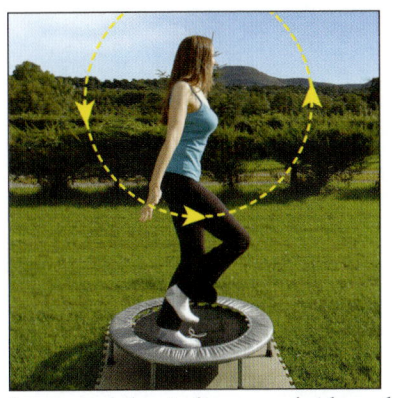

Jogging whilst circling arms backwards

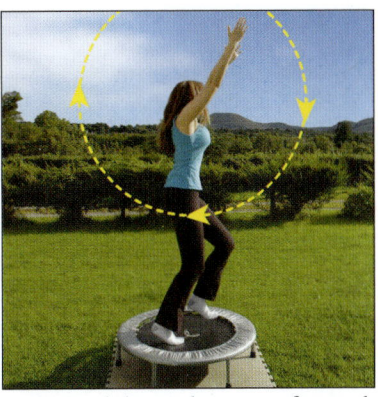

Jogging whilst circling arms forwards

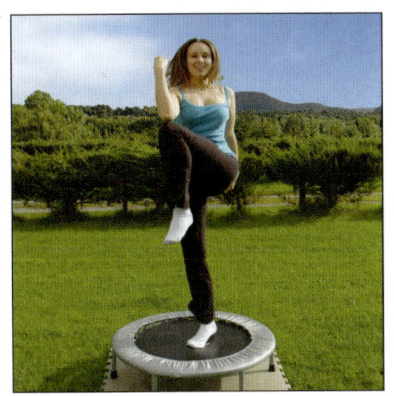

Opposite elbow to knee.

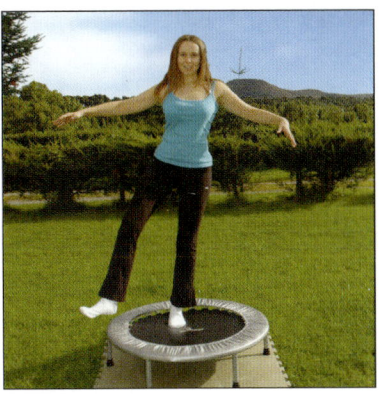

Giving arms and legs a good shake out.

Now, without taking a rest go straight into what I call The Energising Eight. They are eight yoga movements and postures that stretch and tone the whole body, whilst drawing in energy from above and below and from horizontal directions. Be sure to move directly from one posture to the next without any rest, all breathing should be done in and out through the nose, breathing deep into the lower abdomen. This can take a little time to perfect.

THE SUN SALUTATIONS - This is a continuous flow and counted as one of The Energising Eight. Repeat 3 times.

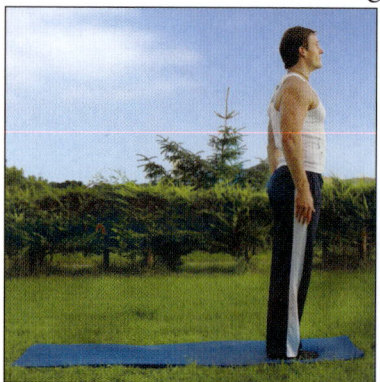

1. Standing erect and aligned.

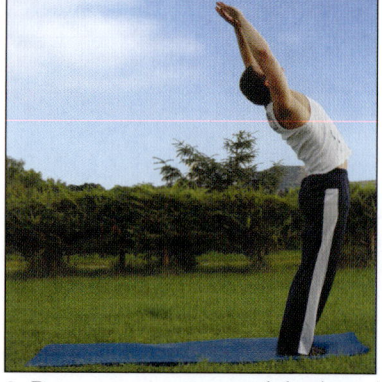

2. Bring arms up & stretch backwards

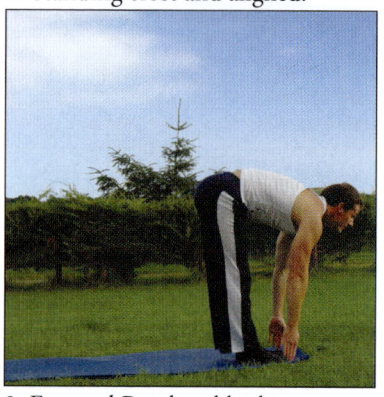

3. Forward Bend and look up.

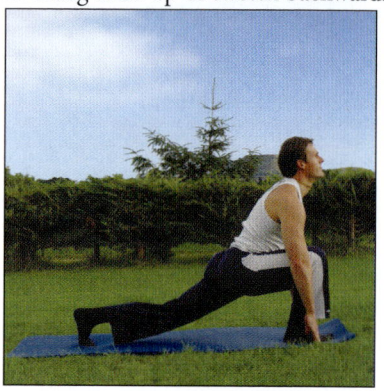

4. Step leg backwards onto toe.

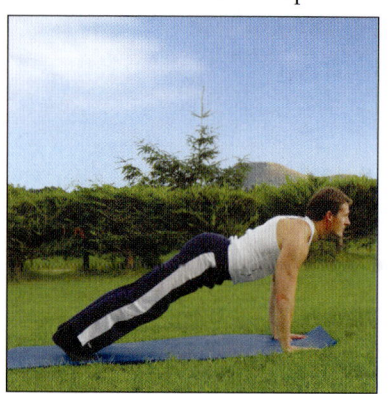

5. Step other leg back, body straight.

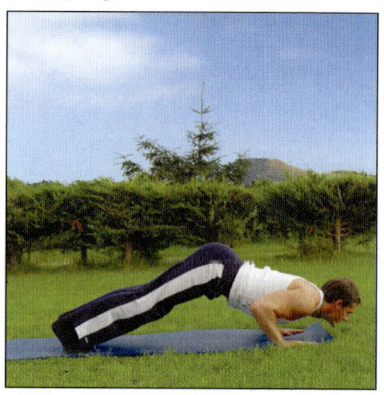

6. Bring upper body down slowly.

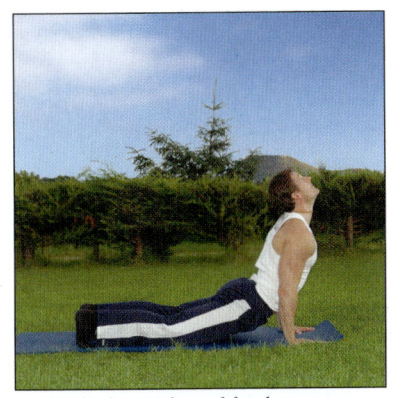

7. Push through and look up

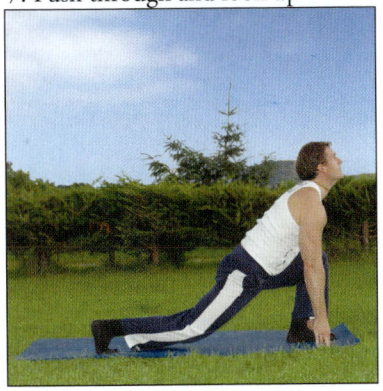

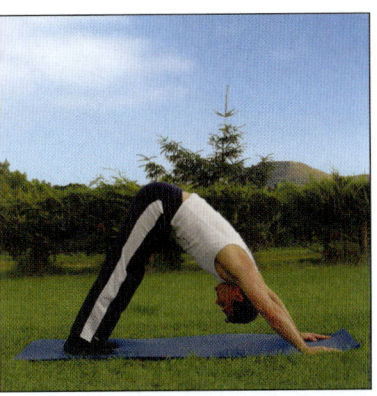

8. Push arms and lift hips backwards.

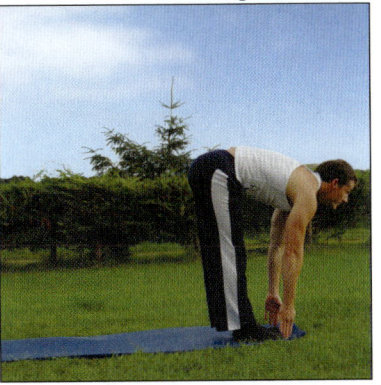

9. Step leg back up between hands.

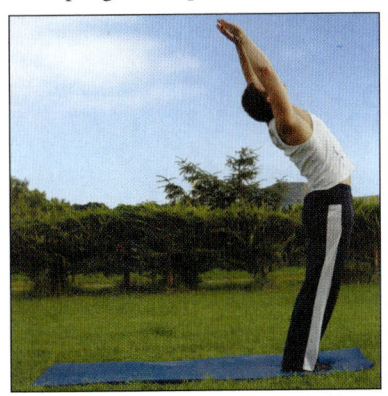

10. Step other leg up & look forward.

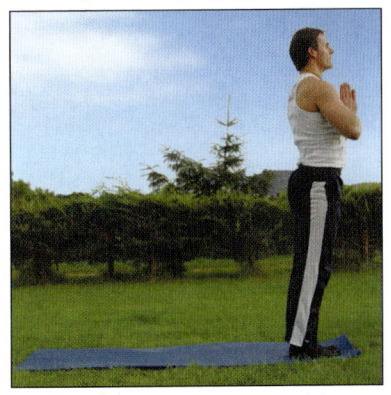

11. Bring arms up & stretch backwards

12. Finish erect in prayer position.

THE WARRIOR POSTURES - Repeat each of the next seven postures on both sides. Hold each posture for seven breaths.

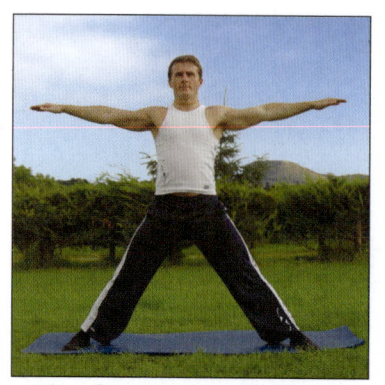

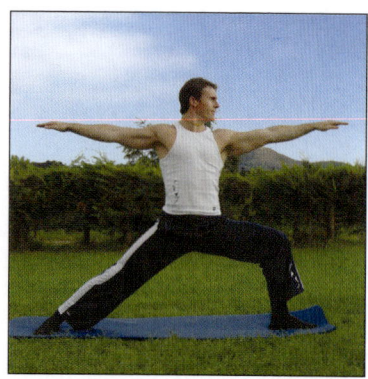

2. Turn foot and head 90 degrees and bend forward knee.

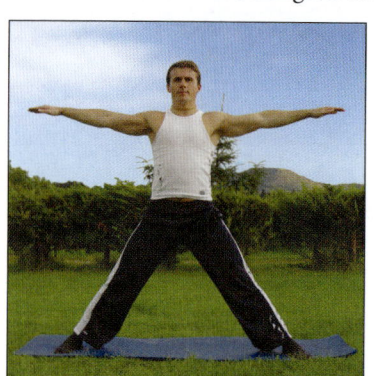

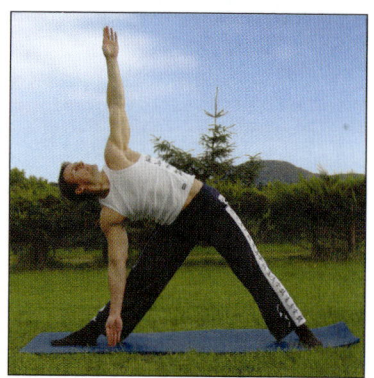

3. Turn foot and head 90 degrees, reach forward and look upwards.

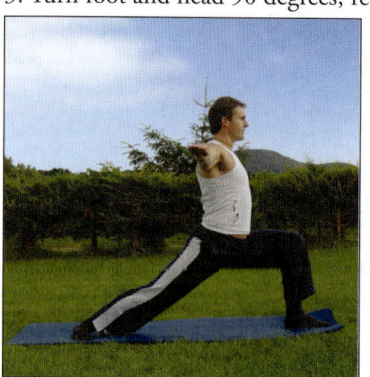

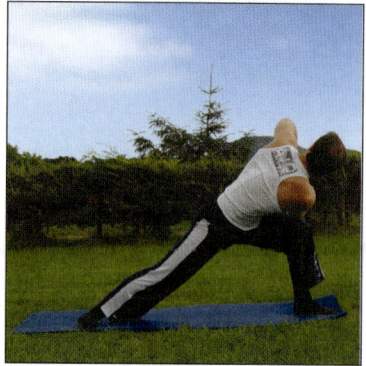

4. Twist placing elbow on opposite knee, hands in prayer position.

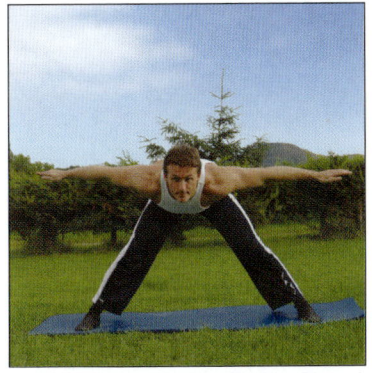

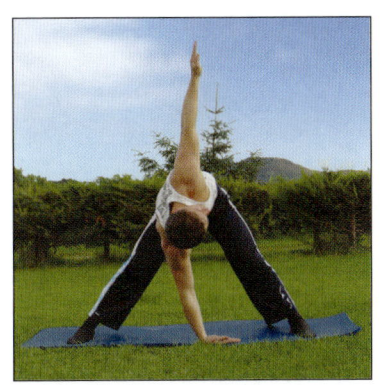

5. Twist body placing back of hand on ground and look upwards.

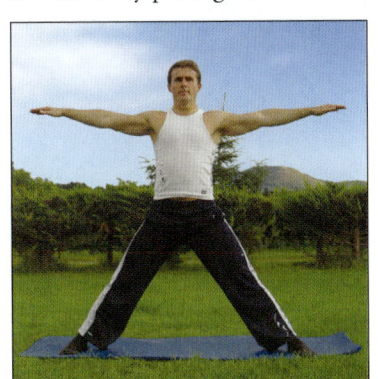

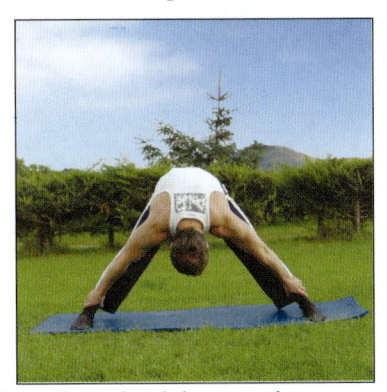

6. Bend forward at waist, grasp both ankles and ease head downwards.

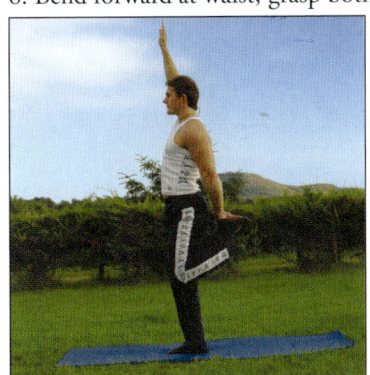

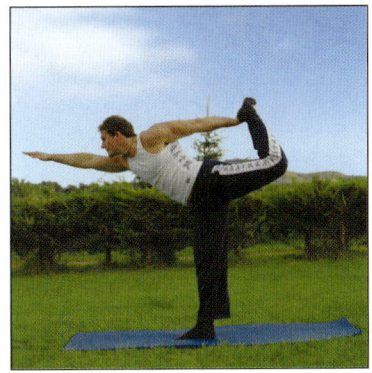

7. Grab inside of raised foot and cant forward arching leg upwards.

105

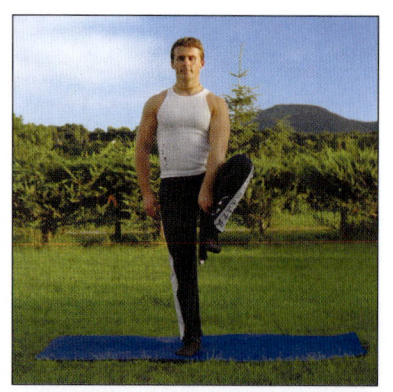

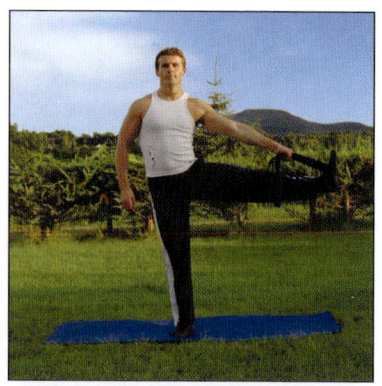

8. Basic Version - Using strap find balance and straighten leg outwards.

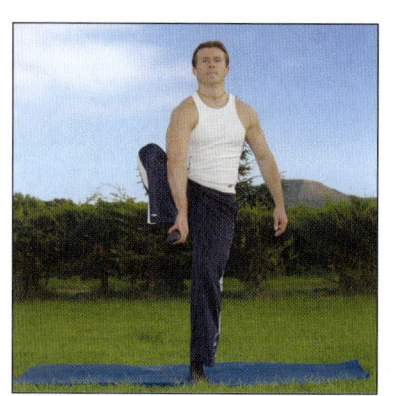

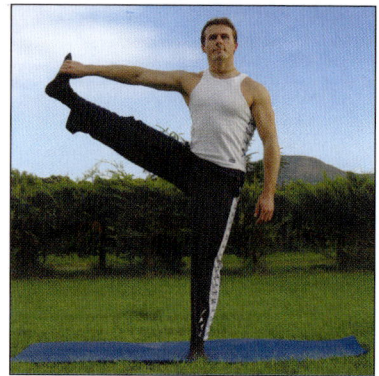

8. Advanced Version - Grasp foot, find balance and straighten leg outwards.

Now from The Energising Eight move straight into the resistance training using the ball. Each exercise is done for 30 seconds and this can be increased up to one minute. Do each movement in a slow and controlled manner,

The Swiss Ball

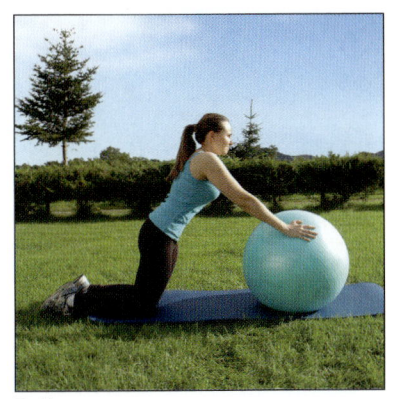

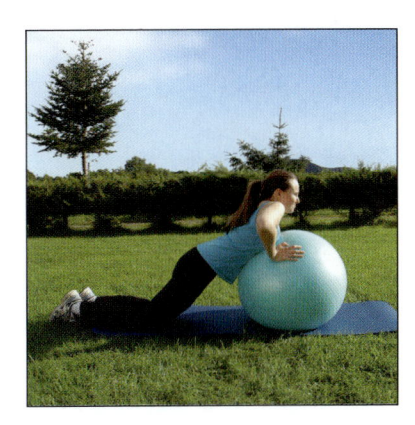

Ball pressups

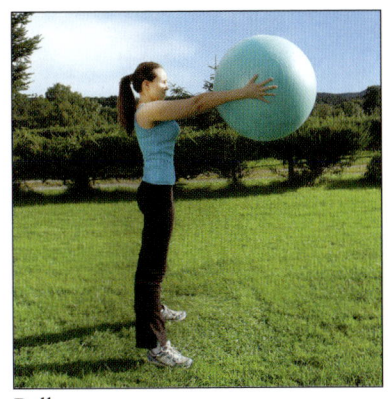

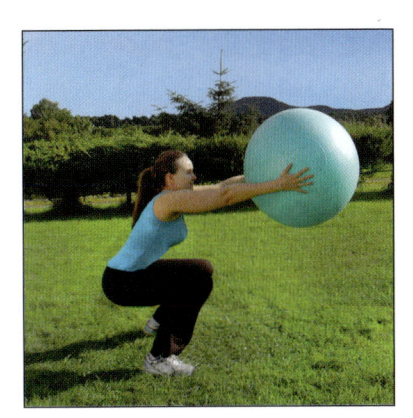

Ball squats

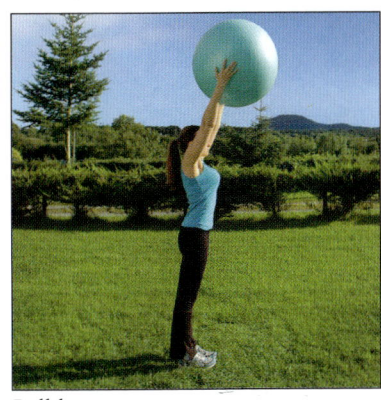

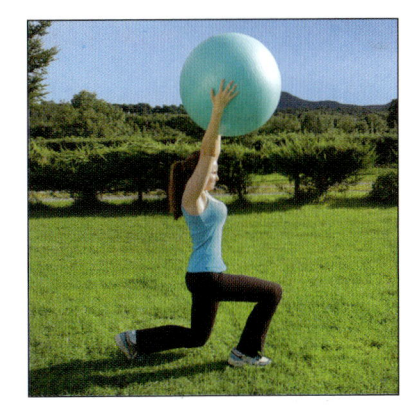

Ball lunges

The Swiss Ball continued...

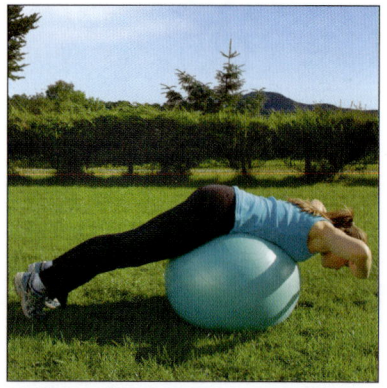

Ball Goodmornings

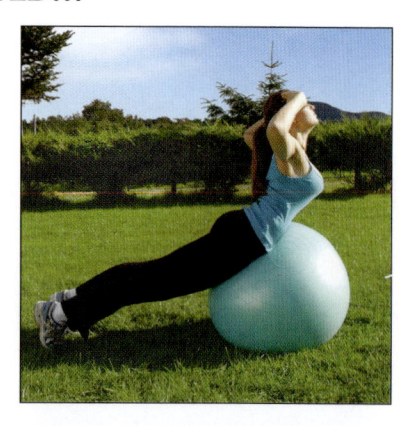

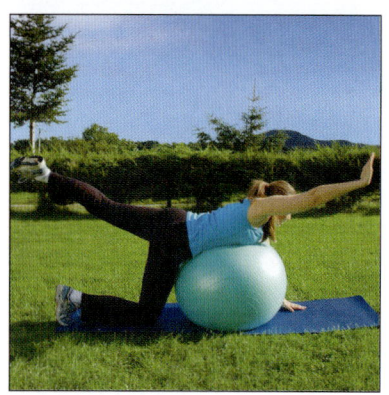

Ball Alternate lifts

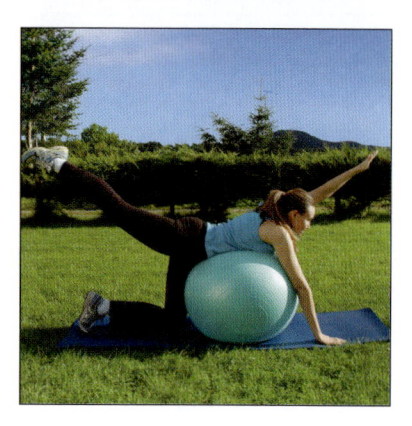

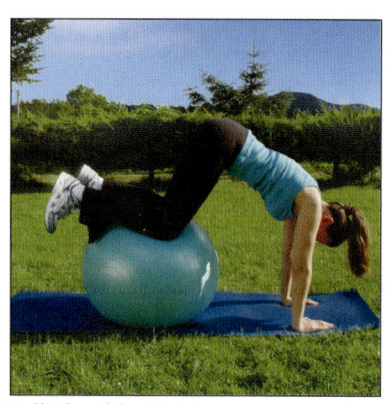

Ball Shoulder Press

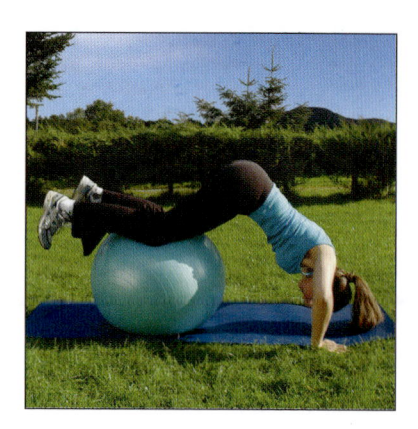

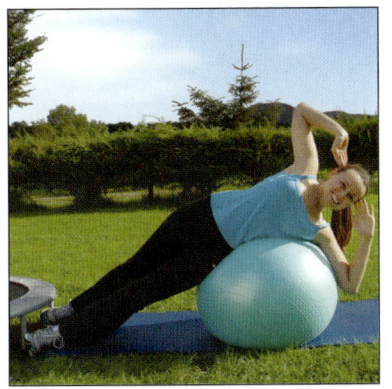

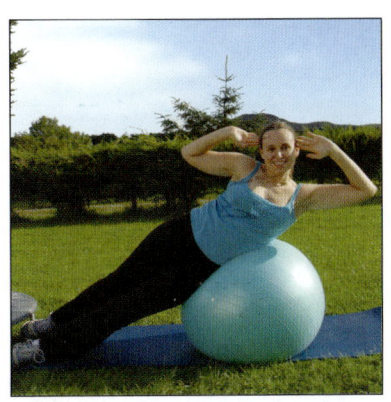

Ball Obliques – Notice feet supported on rebounder. (30 seconds per side)

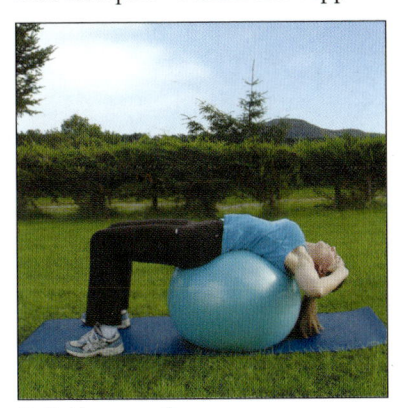

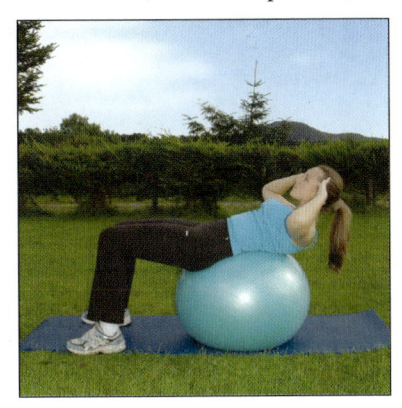

Ball Abs crunch

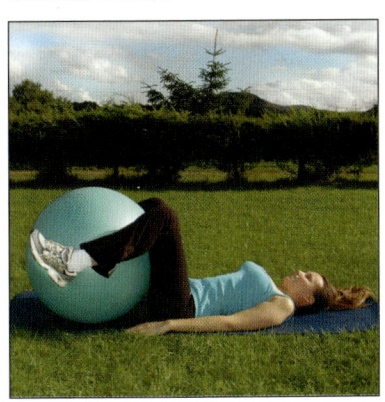

Abs Ball Lift

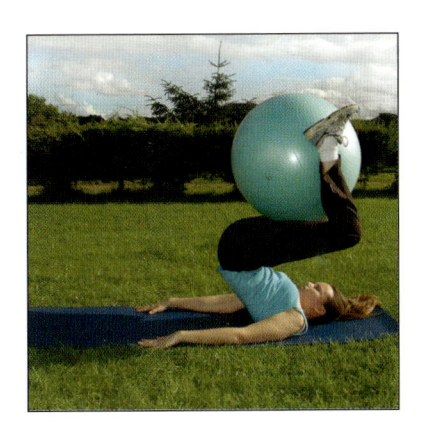

Ki Movements

Now we move onto some stretches that will also allow you to slow down your breathing and rest your muscles. Take two minutes to go through these three movements.

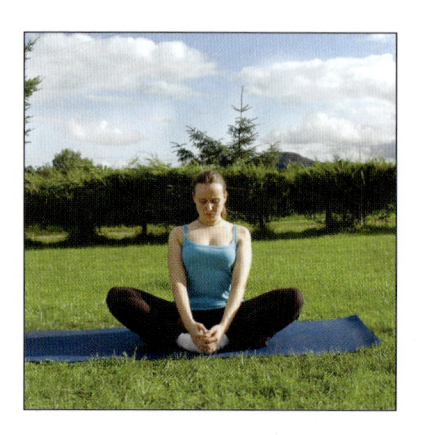

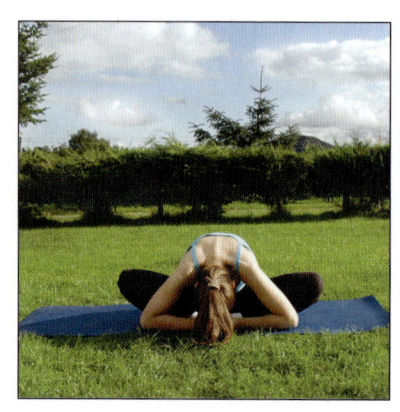

Move the head down towards the toes whilst breathing out and repeat 3 times in total.

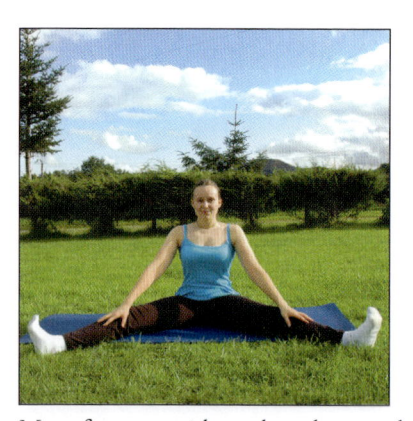

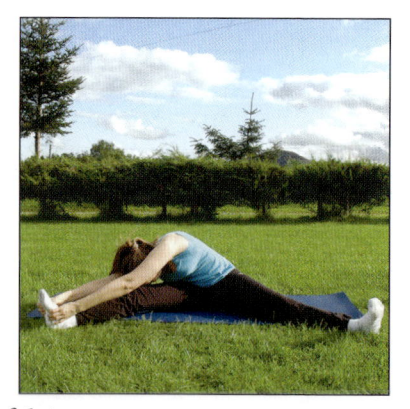

Move from one side to the other, total of 6 times.

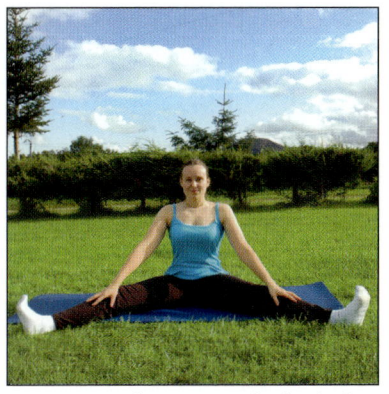

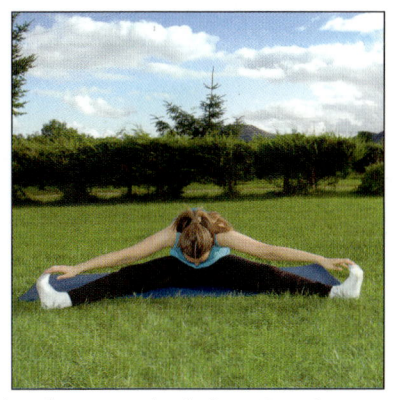

Sitting upright moving the body forward and grasping both feet. Breathe out whilst moving forward. Repeat a total of 3 times.

At this point you will be rested and stretched at the same time and ready for the next two exercises. Now do them immediately.

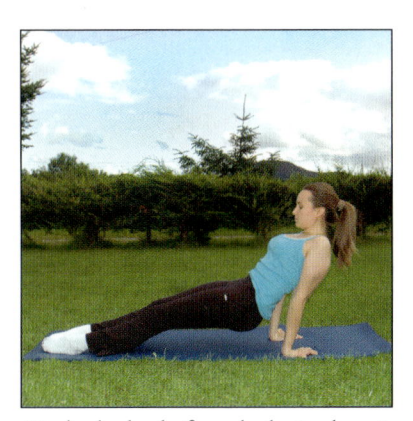

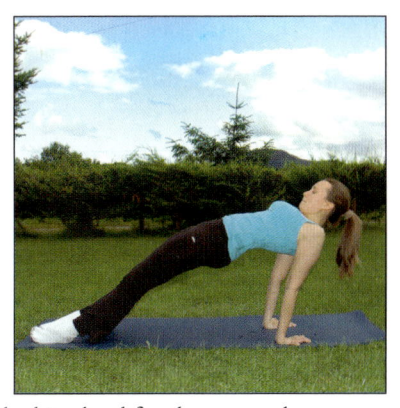

Circle the body first clockwise keeping the hips level for three complete motions, and then anti-clockwise for three motions. Make the circles as slow, controlled and big as possible. Each circle should take 20 seconds, with the whole exercise taking 2 minutes. You can build up to this at it is a difficult exercise and at the same time unbelievably beneficial.

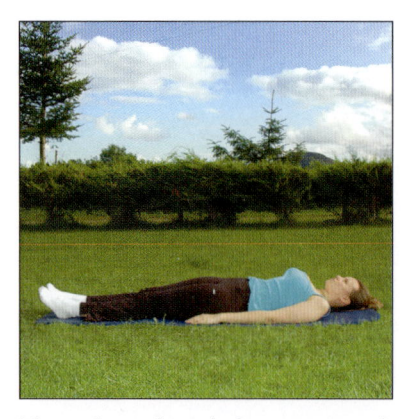

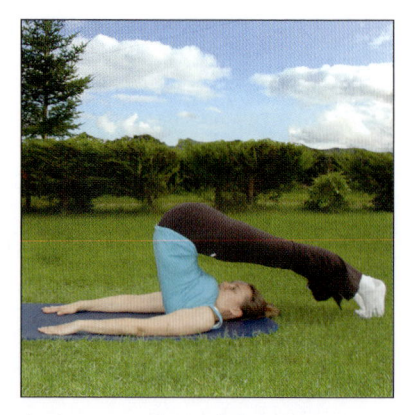

Throughout this whole movement, keep the legs straight and the palms on the ground. As your strength and flexibility increases you will be able to complete the full exercise. It should take 30 seconds for one full repetition. Do six repetitions taking 3 minutes in total.

The workout will finish with the three exercises that were performed after the ball exercises. Remember!

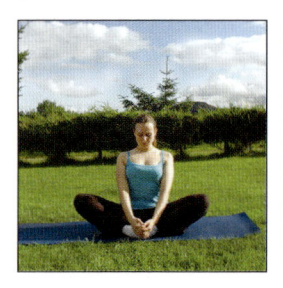

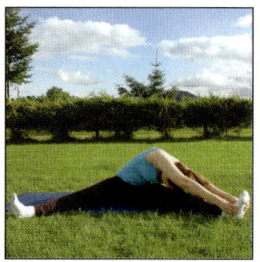

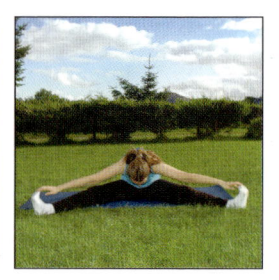

You have completed the CPCS thirty minute workout. A completely transformational physical training system, and you haven't even left your house!

By doing this instead of going to the gym, or some form of exercise class, how much money have you saved on fuel, parking, gym fees and class costs. And how must time have you saved as well. Long term you will actually save yourself years.

Now for Routine Two CPCS.

Apparatus Needed: Pull up bar, dip bar, bar bell, rebounder, Swiss ball.

Like on routine one, the first five minutes is spent warming up on the rebounder. And then it is straight into the energising eight. The Energising Eight should take roughly eight minutes to complete. We then move straight into doing the four most compound strengthening exercises there are.

Do each one after the other without taking a break. If you find you can easily complete twelve repetitions without exhausting the muscles, then either increase the weight up to a maximum of your own body weight, or make the exercise more intense by slowing it down and utilising more control when performing it. Be sure to focus on what you are doing whilst you are doing it. Focus on the muscles being worked, see them getting stronger and more powerful and bring up the images of your body transforming into what you desire it to be.

Pullups

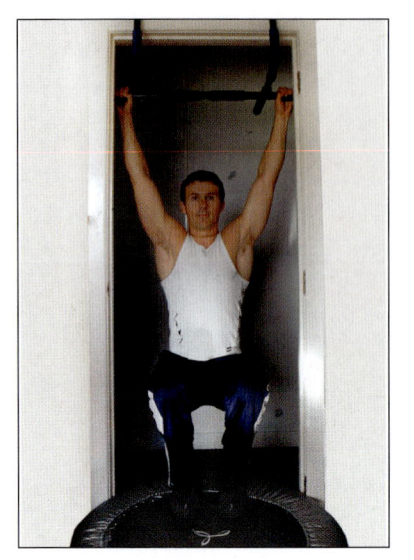

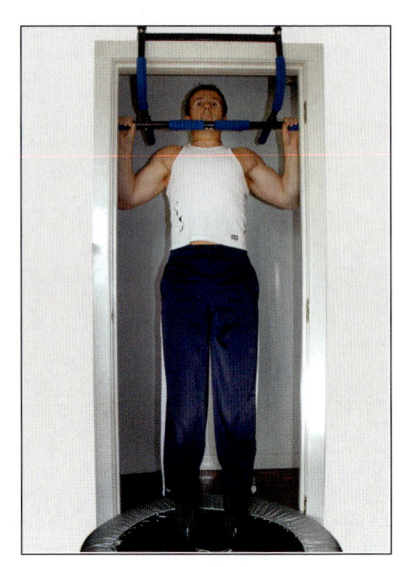

Basic Version – Legs supported on raised platform.

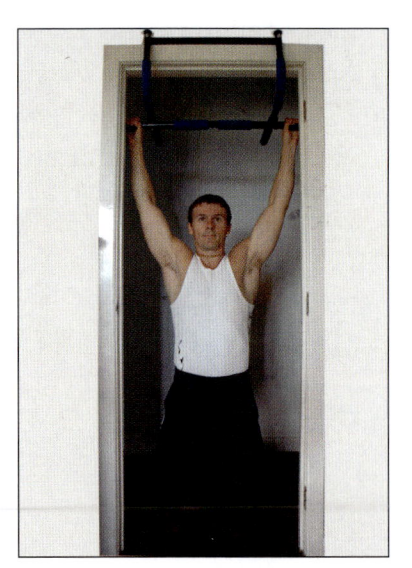

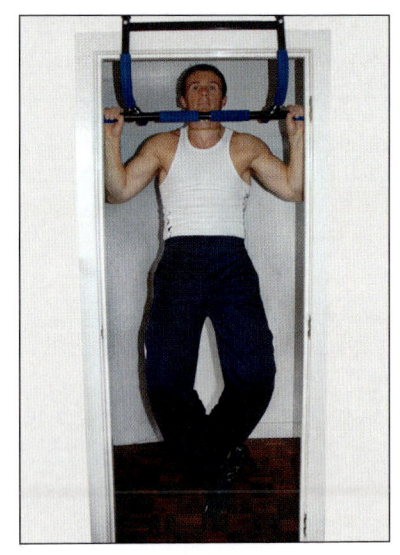

Advanced Version – Pulling up full body weight with arms.

Dips

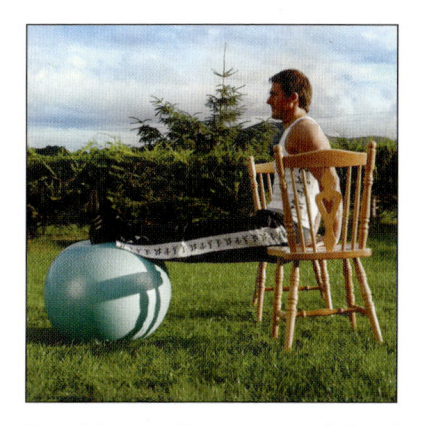

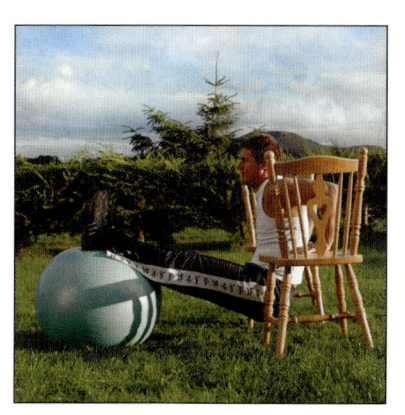

Basic Version - Legs supported. Bend arms 90 degrees then straighten.

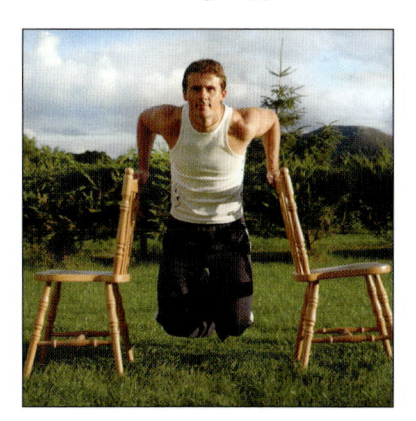

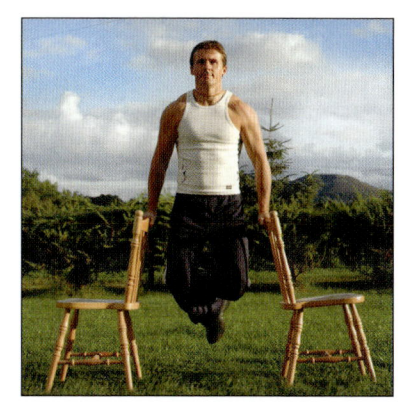

Advanced Version - Body weight fully supported on arms, bend & stretch.

These are great compound exercises, which utilise your own body weight to perform. We call them compound because a few muscle groups are being worked throughout the one motion.

SQUATS FRONT

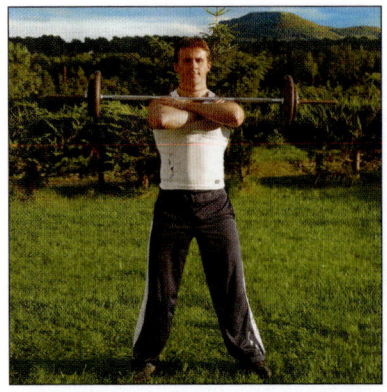

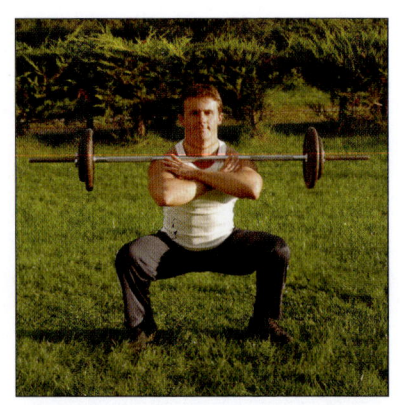

To get the barbell onto your shoulders lift it off the ground with an overhand grip, curl it up to shoulder height, rest it on your shoulders and cross your arms over. This takes practice.

LIFE LIFT WITH SHRUG

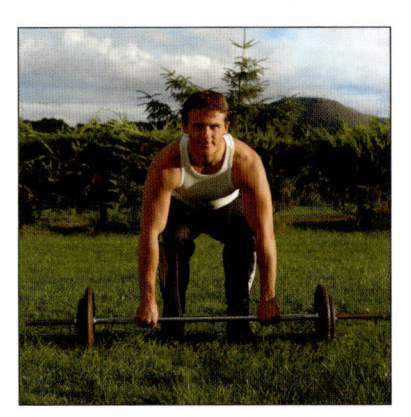

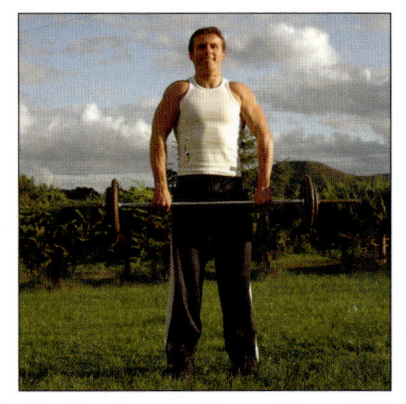

Keep arms straight and weight close to body. Stand up totally straight and lift your shoulders to your ears, back and around. Lower weight slowly to ground and repeat. If you find 12 repetitions easy, then increase the weight you are lifting and also increase the intensity by slowing the movement down and utilising more control.

Remember the three stretches from routine 1? Now do them for 2 minutes.

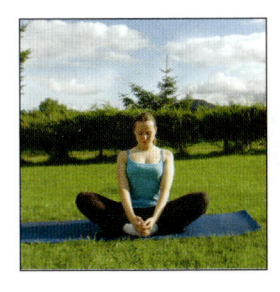

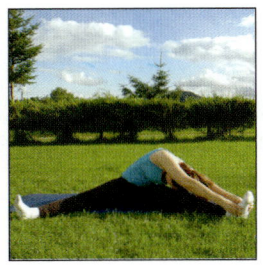

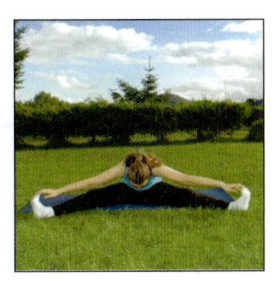

Depending on where you are at physically you can now do this weights and resistance routine again performing the four exercises and then the three stretches. Do it a maximum of three times!

We now finish the routine with these mid-section exercises.

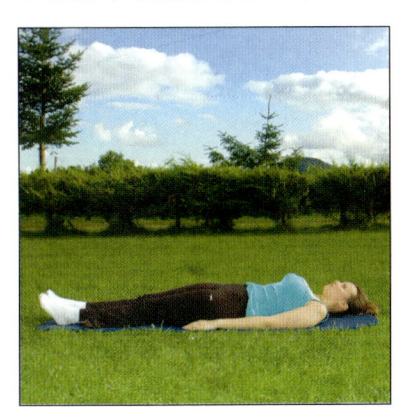

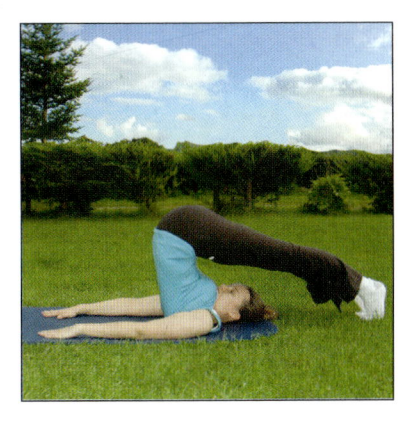

Keep the legs straight throughout. This exercise is to be performed very slowly and controlled for three minutes and you should complete 6 repetitions in total.

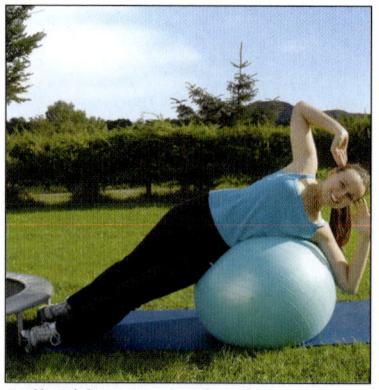

Ball Obliques – both sides.

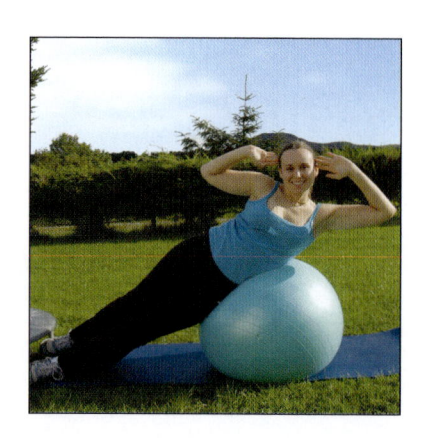

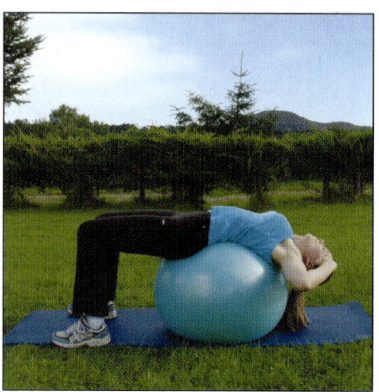

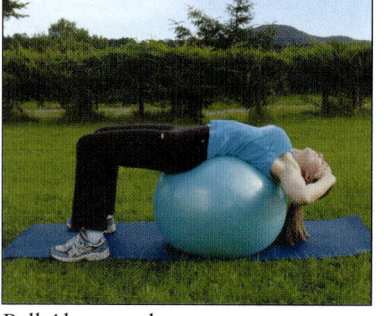

Ball Abs crunch

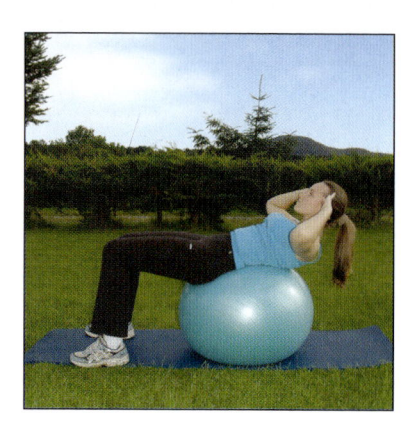

Well done again, you have now completed routine two of the CPCS. Even if you haven't physically done it yet. You have just completed it in your mind as you read through and that is a big step in the right direction.

Routine one is for everybody, and routine two is for those who want to look like an Olympic athlete! As it won't just tone your muscles, it will also build them and build you a strong athletic structure.

I recommend doing each routine for three months and then switch to the other, and keep switching back and forth. This will prevent stagnation with the routines and give you the variety you need.

If the routines look daunting to you right now, that is okay. Take baby steps. Start off by purchasing your new rebounder today! And for the first week just bounce on that. Then add four postures from The Energising Eight the next week, and each week add something else.

You can do this, I know you can. I just heard the other day, that a seventy six year old man recently climbed to the summit of Mount Everest. You know your ABC's right? It's now time to learn your CBA's!

If you can Conceive it, and you can Believe it, then you can Achieve it. This is a truth that our education system neglected to teach.

What can you do with the faith of a mustard seed? That's right! Move a mountain. And I bet you don't weigh quite as much as a mountain, so start moving!

Start the momentum by buying the rebounder and the swiss ball and schedule your daily workouts. Do it now! Show your brain that you are serious. You aren't kidding around any longer. You are a warrior. Your unconscious mind is over 30,000 times more powerful than your conscious mind. This means that you are 30,000 times more powerful than you think you are!

Expand your thinking. You are the most magnificent, powerful and intelligent specimen in this known existence. You are literally capable of anything you decide on. Make some powerful decisions today of where your life is going from now on. No more excuses, no more bullshit. You are now an unstoppable freight train blasting anything that tries to get in your way. It is now time to celebrate. Put on your favourite piece of music and celebrate your existence, your beauty, your passion, your love, your faith, your belief, your joy, your kindness, your honesty, your integrity, your commitment, your unreasonableness, and your power. Because whoever you thought you were before you picked up this book, you now know different. As you read over this small list, and you resonate with each attribute and you know that you are all this and more, and much more. Be Your Potential, because you are it! You are limitless, open up to this concept. Follow your bliss, you cannot wait a second longer. Breathe it in, breathe deeply, and know that you are a Joyous, Everlasting, Divine Individual. This is TRUTH.

Pay it forward

What you have received my friend, I invite you to pay it forward. Giving and receiving is a powerful universal law. This energy must flow, and you can be a part of this cooperative flow of energy by giving three copies of this book to anyone you think could benefit from it. I imagine if someone gave you this book, maybe someone did! How grateful you would be, or how grateful you are to that person. Give three people the gift of this book as you have experienced the gift. You can even take it a step further and set up a group where you can each support each other through the various processes within the book. And even do your workouts together. Share your love by sharing your knowledge.

Order now online at **www.bethinfeelgreat.net**

Receive 20% discount when ordering three or more copies.

Something fundamentally important to your success.

We're not quite finished yet. What I'm going to share with you here is the componant which will ensure your success in all three areas of this book. Without this, making the necessary changes to your life could be a real struggle. Yet, with this knowledge applied, it will be close to easy.

So my question is...Who do you spend your time with? And what are their lifestyle habits? Are your friends positive and optimistic? Do they work out and take care of their body? And do they follow a sound balanced and healthy nutritional plan. If the answer is yes to all these, then that's great. Keep spending time with these people. If you are finding it hard to tick any of the above relating to your friends and the people you spend your time with, then it will be a good idea to start attracting new people into your life who are of this mindset and way of being.

You will find them in health clubs, yoga classes, gyms, and health food stores. Many of the people that you will find in such places are on the same path as you, and will encourage and support you in your dreams and desires. When you go for lunch with them, they won't bring you to the local fast food outlet and insist you go for the dessert when you are obviously full.

You see there are two revolutions going on at the moment. There is a health revolution and a fat revolution. Both are doing well and have excellent campaigns running. It is you who must decide which one you would like to be a part of. Which one will serve you at your highest level. You know the answer, I don't need to tell you.

Now for a story. Remember it well and apply the message to all areas of your life.

There once was a farmer, and it was time for the farmer to plough his land. For this task the farmer had two donkeys. Over time the donkeys had become fat and lazy and they refused to plough the land. They preferred to eat grass all day and lay about under the shade of the trees.

Fed up with his fat, lazy donkeys, the farmer went to the local market and asked the donkey salesman for his most motivated and hardest working donkey. The donkey salesman brings the farmer his prize donkey and tells him that there never was a more hard working donkey than the one he was giving him. Happy the farmer returns home and starts ploughing his land with his new donkey. The other two donkeys laughed and sniggered at the new donkey and every time he passed with the plough, they would say *"Hey what are you doing working so hard in the hot sun? It's nice and comfortable here in the shade and there's lots of grass to eat."*

After only a few days of spending time with the other two donkeys, the new donkey had started to take on their habits and character traits. The farmer, no matter how hard he tried could not get the donkey to work. The donkey preferred to laze under the shade of the trees and eat grass all day.

The farmer, now angry at the lazy donkey he had been given, returns him to the donkey salesman and demands a new donkey. *"But this is my finest donkey"* protests the donkey salesman. *"He refuses to work, I need a real working donkey"*, demands the farmer. *"As you wish sir"*, says the donkey salesman taking his donkey back and giving the farmer his second finest donkey. Happy, the farmer returns to the farm and puts the donkey to work ploughing the fields.

Again, the fat lazy donkeys tease the new donkey about all the hard work she is doing, and how life is much easier and more comfortable for them. After only a few days, spending time with the donkeys, the new donkey has taken on their beliefs and habits and refuses to work. The farmer, furious at how he has been conned a second time, brings the donkey back to the salesman and rants about how both donkeys that he bought are just as lazy as his own donkeys and want to do nothing but spend time in the shade eating grass with his fat, lazy donkeys. *"Aha"*, says the donkey salesman, nodding with a look of knowing on his face. *"The problem is not with my donkeys"*, he says. *"Then what is it"*? Says the farmer, clearly frustrated.

"Let me put it this way", says the donkey salesman. *"Show me the people you spend your time with, and I will show you your life"*

Transformational Coaching

How would you like to have the opportunity to work personally with me or one of my highly trained coaches? Well, I am offering you that opportunity right now!

A coach will help you make rapid progress in your life, accelerating you directly towards the achievement of your goals. A coach will be objective and honest with you so that you realise your potential letting self imposed obstacles dissolve away.

A coach will assist you in creating an empowering identity for yourself that will make motivation effortless. A coach will hold you accountable, so every week you know you must take those actions or you will have your coach asking you why not at the end of the week.

A coach will hold you to a higher standard than anyone else will, and be encouraging and supportive when challenges arise. This is just the tip of the iceberg of what you will get when you hire a transformational coach. You truly are making a commitment to yourself.

Go ahead and make that leap. You deserve it! Visit **www.bethinfeelgreat.net** now.

A final blessing

There is an amazing power in blessings. One of the greatest gifts you can give a person is to bless them. Anyone can bless another as long as they themselves feel blessed.

A blessing comes deep from a persons soul and can heal and transform the person who is being blessed!

To feel blessed, you must cultivate appreciation within yourself. Start off general by appreciating life, the sun, the moon, the stars, the earth, the water, the trees and then bring your focus to more specific things in your day to day life. Your health, your family, friends, a roof over your head, a bed to sleep in, running water and food to eat, to start with. Make this a daily ritual and you will begin to feel so blessed, and then you can bless others and assist in their healing and transformation.

Take a few moments right now to close you eyes and realise and feel how blessed you truly are.

About the Author

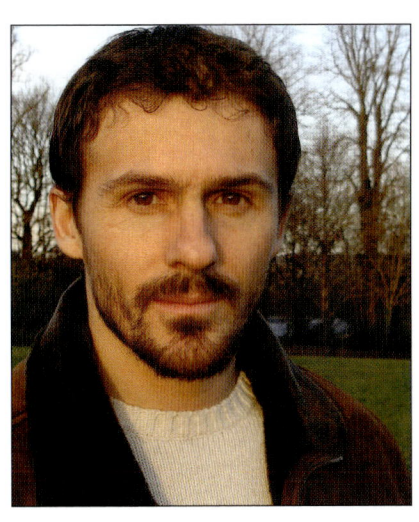

Matthew Armstrong's quest began at age seven, when he started training in Martial Arts. He now holds an 8th dan black belt in Japanese Arts and a 2nd degree black sash in Chinese Arts.

At eighteen he joined the Royal Marines Commandos and completed a five year service in which he became a reconaissance leader, and received a commendation for courage under fire.

He has circumnavigated the globe many times over, devoting his time to studying with many of the worlds great wizards. Including Martial Arts Masters, Spiritual Masters, Taoist Healing Masters, Yoga Guru's, Olympic Trainers, Natural Health Experts and World Thought Leaders.

His driving force being to learn, grow and then contribute this integrated knowledge of what he has absorbed and who he has become in the process.

The message he brings is that of transformation, with his mission being to educate, inspire and ultimately transform the lives of those who are ready and willing to step up!

He is the founder and CEO of Be Your Potential, which offers coaching, training and speaking services.

Also available 2009...

Preorder Now! @ www.beyourpotential.net

You Will stop smoking and feel great

This is the second book in the "You Will Feel Great" series, and is like no other book out there on the subject of smoking cessation.

It goes beyond dealing with the behavior to zeroing in on the route issue, which will give lasting results.

To ensure success there is an exclusive members website, which includes audios and videos that really help the individual to completely free themselves of this life debilitating and killer habit.

My driving force to write this book was watching my auntie slowly suffocate to death during a period of over a decade. Unable to leave the house for the last five years, and on a constant supply of oxygen and inhalers and knowing that the cause was smoking.

She wanted to know that her pain was not in vain. No one should have to go through this, so take action now if you or anyone you know and care about smokes then you need this book. It will change you life and move you towards the light.

You Will Be Young Again and Feel Great

Preorder Now! @ www.beyourpotential.net

How would you like to live past your 100th birthday with energy and vitality?

No matter what your age, you must start now.

In this book you will learn everything you need to reverse your biological clock and become perpetually young.

Pain and dis-ease will become a thing of the past as you become limber, flexible strong, youthful and feel all the great emotions of excitement, joy and happiness that go along with that.

Prepare to transform your mind and body to how you should be.

As well as the book you will receive access to a free exclusive members website, which included audios and videos to educate and inspire you along on your journey to becoming young again.

Be Thin Feel Great Retreat

Come and join us on a "Be Thin Feel Great" Retreat. The normal price for a six day retreat is £1995. When you book your place and produce this ticket, you will receive a £1498 discount.

Two retreats are held every year and a maximum of 25 people are accepted onto each retreat, which keeps it intimate and personal and makes sure that everyone is served.

BE THIN FEEL GREAT RETREAT

This ticket allows you the special price of £497 for the full six day retreat.

Ticket Value: - £1498

Priority Code: 17091976

At the completion of the retreat you will be physically, mentally, emotionally and spiritually TRANSFORMED.

Book your place now @ **www.bethinfeelgreat.net**